DSM-IV-TR
Handbook
of
Differential
Diagnosis

DSM-IV-TR
Handbook
of
Differential
Diagnosis

Michael B. First, M.D.
Allen Frances, M.D.
Harold Alan Pincus, M.D.

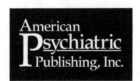

American Psychiatric Publishing, Inc.

Washington, DC
London, England

Note: The authors have worked to ensure that all information in this book concerning drug dosages, schedules, and routes of administration is accurate as of the time of publication and consistent with standards set by the U.S. Food and Drug Administration and the general medical community. As medical research and practice advance, however, therapeutic standards may change. For this reason and because human and mechanical errors sometimes occur, we recommend that readers follow the advice of a physician who is directly involved in their care or the care of a member of their family.

Copyright © 2002 American Psychiatric Publishing, Inc.
ALL RIGHTS RESERVED
Manufactured in the United States of America on acid-free paper
06 05 04 03 02   5 4 3 2 1
First Edition

American Psychiatric Publishing, Inc.
1400 K Street, N.W.
Washington, DC 20005
www.appi.org

Library of Congress Cataloging-in-Publication Data
First, Michael B., 1956–
    DSM-IV-TR handbook of differential diagnosis / Michael B. First, Allen Frances, Harold Alan Pincus.
        p.   cm.
    Includes bibliographical references and index.
    ISBN 1-58562-054-8 (pbk. : alk. paper)
    1. Mental illness—Diagnosis—Handbooks, manuals, etc.
    2. Diagnosis, Differential—Handbooks, manuals, etc. I. Frances, Allen, 1942–   . II. Pincus, Harold Alan, 1951–   . III. Title.
    [DNLM: 1. Mental Disorders—diagnosis. 2. Diagnosis, Differential. 3. Mental Disorders—classification.   WM 141 F527d 2002]
    RC473.D54 F553 2002
    616.89′075—dc21

                                                                                2001045808

British Library Cataloguing in Publication Data
A CIP record is available from the British Library.

To our parents:
Reda and David First,
Julia Frances and in memory of Joseph Frances,
and Charlotte Pincus and in memory of Jack Pincus

Contents

Preface

Differential diagnosis is the bread and butter of our task as clinicians. Most patients don't come to the office saying "I have Major Depressive Disorder . . . give me an antidepressant" (although some do!). More typically, the patient consults us with particular symptoms that are the source of clinically significant distress or impairment. Confronted with one (or a couple) of specific symptoms, it is our job to cull from the wide universe of DSM-IV-TR conditions those that could possibly account for them. Once we are armed with this initial list of possibilities, our next job is to collect additional information (from personal history, family history, mental status examination, or laboratory investigations) that will allow a winnowing down of the list to a single "most likely" contender, which becomes the initial diagnosis leading to the initial treatment plan. One must still keep an open mind, however. Confirmation of the initial diagnosis often requires the passage of time so that the telltale features of the course can play themselves out.

This handbook should improve your skill in formulating a comprehensive differential diagnosis by presenting the problem from a number of different perspectives. In Chapter 1, "Differential Diagnosis Step by Step," we explore the differential diagnostic issues that must be considered in each and every patient being evaluated. In Chapter 2, "Differential Diagnosis by the Trees," we approach differential diagnosis from the bottom up—that is, a point of origin that begins with the patient's presenting symptom(s). Each of the 27 decision trees indicates which DSM-IV-TR diagnoses must be considered in the differential diagnosis of that particular symptom and outlines the thinking process involved in choosing from among the possible contenders. In Chapter 3, "Differential Diagnosis by the Tables," we approach differential diagnosis from a later point in the assessment process—that is, once you have reached a tentative diagnosis and want to ensure that all reasonable alternatives have received adequate consideration. This section contains 62 differential diagnostic tables, one for each of the most important DSM-IV-TR disorders. Chapter 4, "DSM-IV-TR Symptom Index," includes a symptom index that lists in a convenient form those disorders that one should think of when formulating a differential diagnosis given a particular symptom in the patient's presentation. Finally, the handbook closes with the DSM-IV-TR Classification, which has been included to facilitate coding and to provide an overview of all of the diagnoses that must be considered in differential diagnosis.

The information provided in the decision trees, the differential diagnosis tables, and the symptom index is somewhat overlapping, but each format also has its own strengths and may be more or less useful depending on the situation. The decision trees highlight the overall algorithmic rules that govern the classification of a particular symptom. In contrast, the symptom index does not indicate any of the rules of association but does offer the greatest level of specificity by covering a wider range of presenting symptoms. The differential diagnostic tables have the advantage of providing a head-to-head comparison of each disorder and its nearest neighbors. Different readers will have different purposes and different methods of using this handbook. Some individuals will be interested in a comprehensive overview of psychiatric diagnosis and will find it rewarding to review the handbook cover to cover. Others will use the handbook more as a reference guide to assist in the differential diagnosis of a particular patient.

The art and science of psychiatric diagnosis is both cursed and blessed by the fact that individuals are ever so much more complex than the information laid out in any set of decision trees, tables, and indices. One must always temper the temptation to apply DSM-IV-TR or this handbook in a rote or cookbook fashion. The approaches outlined here are meant to enhance and not to replace the central role of clinical judgment and the wisdom of accumulated experience. On the other hand, clinicians who are not aware of the guidelines for differential diagnosis included in DSM-IV-TR may become idiosyncratic in their diagnostic and treatment habits. It is useful to know and use DSM-IV-TR but not be enslaved by it.

Differential Diagnosis
Step by Step

The process of differential diagnosis can be broken down into six basic steps: 1) ruling out Malingering/Factitious Disorder, 2) ruling out a substance etiology, 3) ruling out an etiological general medical condition, 4) determining the specific primary disorder(s), 5) differentiating Adjustment Disorder from Not Otherwise Specified (NOS), and 6) establishing the boundary with no mental disorder. A thorough review of this chapter provides a useful framework for understanding and applying the decision trees presented in the next chapter.

Step 1: Is the Presenting Symptom for Real?

We include this as our first step because it is so often missed in clinical practice. Most of our work depends on a good faith collaborative effort between the clinician and the patient to uncover the nature and cause of the presenting symptoms. There are times, however, when everything may not be as it seems. Some patients may elect to deceive the clinician by producing or feigning the presenting symptoms. Others may elaborate symptoms through mechanisms that are outside of their conscious awareness. There are two conditions in DSM-IV-TR that are characterized by conscious feigning— Malingering and Factitious Disorder—and one by unconscious feigning— Conversion Disorder. Malingering and Factitious Disorder are differentiated based on the motivation for the conscious deception. When the motivation for the behavior is the achievement of a clearly recognizable goal (e.g., insurance compensation, avoiding legal or military responsibilities, obtaining drugs), this is considered Malingering. When the motivation is the specific need to assume the sick role without obvious external gain, then a diagnosis of Factitious Disorder is more likely. Unconscious feigning can occur in suggestible individuals as a means of solving conflicts, validating their inability to function, and seeking help. Whereas historically most such patients presented to neurological settings with "neurological" presentations (i.e., Conversion Disorder), currently such individuals are more likely to present to psychiatric settings with psychiatric presentations (e.g., the apparent rise in the incidence of Dissociative Identity Disorder).

We are certainly not advocating that the every patient should be treated as a hostile witness and that every clinician should become a cynical district attorney. However, the clinician's index of suspicion should be raised 1) in situations in which feigning of symptoms is relatively common (e.g., emergency rooms, forensic hearings, prisons, inpatient hospitals), 2) when the patient presents with a cluster of psychiatric symptoms that conforms more to a lay perception of mental illness rather than to a recognized clinical entity, 3) when the nature of the symptoms shifts radically from one clinical encounter to another, 4) when the patient has a presentation that mimics that of a role model (e.g., another patient on the unit), and 5) when the patient is manipulative or suggestible. Finally, it is useful for clinicians to become mindful of tendencies they might have toward being either excessively skeptical or excessively gullible.

Step 2: Rule Out Substance Etiology (Including Drugs of Abuse, Medication, Toxin Exposure)

The first question that should always be considered in differential diagnosis is whether the presenting symptoms arise from a substance that is exerting a direct effect on the central nervous system (CNS).   Virtually any presentation that is encountered in a mental health setting can be caused by substance use. Missing a substance etiology is probably the single most common diagnostic error made in clinical practice. This is particularly unfortunate because a correct diagnosis has immediate treatment implications. For example, if one determines that depressed mood is due to alcohol withdrawal, it usually does not make sense to immediately start an antidepressant medication. The determination of whether psychopathology is due to substance use often can be difficult because, although substance use is fairly ubiquitous and a wide variety of different symptoms can be caused by substances, the fact that substance use and psychopathology occur together does not necessarily imply a cause-and-effect relationship.

Obviously, your first task is to determine if the person has been using a substance.   This entails careful history taking and physical examination for signs of intoxication or withdrawal. Because substance-abusing individuals are notorious for underestimating their intake, it is usually wise to consult with family members and obtain laboratory analysis of body fluids to ascertain the presence of particular substances. It should be remembered that patients who use or are exposed to substances other than drugs of abuse can and often do present with psychiatric symptoms. Medication-induced psychopathology is more and more common, and very often missed, especially as the population ages and many individuals are on multiple medications. Although it is less common, toxin exposure should be considered especially for those whose occupations bring them into contact with potential toxins.

Once the substance use has been established, the next step is to determine whether there is an etiological relationship between it and the psychiatric symptomatology.   This requires distinguishing among three possible relationships between the substance use and the psychopathology: 1) that the psychiatric symptoms result from the direct effects of the substance on the CNS, 2) that the substance use is a consequence (or associated feature) of having a primary psychiatric disorder (e.g., "self-medication"), and 3) that the psychiatric symptoms and the substance use are independent. We begin with a discussion of the first case—what in DSM-IV-TR are called the Substance-Induced Disorders (e.g., Cocaine-Induced Psychotic Disorder, Reserpine-Induced Mood Disorder).

In diagnosing a Substance-Induced Disorder, there are three aspects to determining whether there is a causal relationship between the substance use and the psychiatric symptomatology.   First, you must determine whether there is a close temporal relationship between the substance use and the psychiatric symptoms. Then, you must consider the likelihood that the particular pattern of substance use can result in the observed psychiatric symptoms. Finally, you should consider whether there are better alternative explanations (i.e., nonsubstance induced) for the clinical picture.

The temporal sequence between the substance use and the onset or maintenance of the psychopathology is probably the best (although still fallible) method for evaluating their etiological relationship. At the extremes this is clear-cut. If the onset of the psychopathology clearly precedes the onset of the substance use, then it is likely that a nonsubstance psychiatric condition is primary and the substance use is secondary (e.g., as a form of self-medication) or is unrelated. Conversely, if the onset of the substance use clearly and closely precedes the psychopathology, it lends greater credence to the likelihood of a Substance-Induced Disorder. Unfortunately, in practice this seemingly simple determination can be quite difficult because the onsets of the substance use and the psychopathology may be more or less simultaneous or impossible to reconstruct retrospectively. In such situations, you will have to rely more on what happens when the person no longer takes the substance. Psychiatric symptoms that occur in the context of Substance Intoxication, Substance Withdrawal, and medication use result from the effects of the substance on neurotransmitter systems. Once these effects have been removed (by a period of abstinence after the withdrawal phase), the symptoms should spontaneously resolve. Persistence of the psychiatric symptomatology for a significant period of time beyond periods of intoxication or withdrawal suggests that the psychopathology is primary and not due to substance use. The exceptions to this are Substance-Induced Persisting Dementia and Persisting Amnestic Disorder, in which by definition the cognitive symptoms are due to permanent CNS damage, and not due to the acute effects of substance use, and therefore persist well beyond the usual duration of Substance Intoxication or Withdrawal.

The DSM-IV-TR criteria for substance-induced presentations suggest that psychiatric symptoms be attributed to the substance use if they remit within a month of the cessation of acute intoxication, withdrawal, or medication use. During the DSM-IV deliberations, the choice of a 4-week limit was somewhat controversial, and this guideline must be applied with clinical judgment. Some clinicians, particularly those who work in substance use treatment settings, were most concerned about the possibility of misdiagnosing a substance-induced presentation as a primary mental disorder that is not caused by the substance use. Thus, they suggested allowing 6–8 weeks of abstinence before considering the diagnosis to be a primary mental disorder. On the other hand, those who work primarily in psychiatric settings were concerned that, given the wide use of substances among patients seen in clinical settings, such a long waiting period is impractical and might result in an overdiagnosis of Substance-Induced Disorders and an underdiagnosis of primary mental disorders. Moreover, it must be recognized that any chosen generic time frame would have to apply to a wide variety of substances with very different properties and a wide variety of possibly consequent psychopathologies. Remember, therefore, that the time frame must be applied flexibly, taking into account the extent, duration, and nature of the substance use as noted below. One suggestion was to specify different waiting periods for each class of substance. This interesting proposal was ultimately rejected because there was insufficient evidence to set thresholds for each class of substance, and it would have made the system impossibly complex. On balance, it seems that the 4-week threshold included in DSM-IV (and DSM-IV-TR) provides a useful suggestion for how long after drug use one should wait before making the diagnosis of a primary mental disorder, but a great deal of clinical judgment is required in applying it.

Sometimes, it is simply not possible to determine whether there was a period of time when the psychiatric symptoms occurred outside of periods of substance use. This may occur in the often-encountered situation in which the patient is too poor a historian to allow a careful determination of past temporal relationships. In addition, substance use and psychiatric symptoms can have their onset around the same time (often in adolescence), and both can be more or less chronic and continuous. In these situations, it may be necessary to assess the patient during a current period of abstinence from substance use. If the psychiatric symptoms persist in the absence of substance use, then the psychiatric disorder can be considered to be primary. If the symptoms remit, then the substance use is probably primary. It is important to realize that this judgment can only be made after waiting for enough time to elapse so as to be confident that the psychiatric symptoms are not a consequence of substance withdrawal. Ideally, the best setting for making this determination is in the hospital, where the patient's access to substances can be controlled and the patient's psychiatric symptomatology can be serially assessed. Of course, it is often impossible in this era of brief hospitalizations to observe a patient for as long as 4 weeks in a tightly controlled setting. Consequently, these judgments must be based on less controlled observation, and one's confidence in the accuracy of the diagnosis should be more guarded.

In determining the likelihood that the pattern of substance use can account for the symptoms, you must also consider whether the nature, amount, and duration of substance use are consistent with the pattern of the observed psychiatric symptoms. Only certain substances are known to be causally related to particular psychiatric symptoms. Moreover, the amount of substance taken and duration of its use must be above a certain threshold for it to be considered the cause of the psychiatric symptomatology. For example, a severe and persisting depressed mood following the isolated use of a small amount of cocaine should probably not be considered to be attributed to the cocaine use, even though depressed mood is sometimes associated with cocaine withdrawal.

You should also take into account other factors in the presentation that suggest that the presentation is not caused by a substance. These include a history of many similar episodes not related to substance use, a strong family history of the particular primary disorder, or the presence of physical examination or laboratory findings suggesting that a general medical condition might be involved. Considering factors other than substance use as a cause for the presentation of psychiatric symptoms requires fine clinical judgment (and often waiting and seeing) to weigh the relative probabilities in these situations. For example, an individual may have heavy family loading for anxiety disorders and still have a cocaine-induced panic attack that does not necessarily presage the development of primary Panic Disorder.

In some cases, the substance use can be the consequence or associated feature (rather than the cause) of psychiatric symptomatology.   Not uncommonly, the substance-taking behavior can be considered a form of self-medication for the psychiatric condition. For example, an individual with a primary anxiety disorder might use alcohol excessively for its sedative and antianxiety effects. One interesting implication of using a substance to self-medicate is that individuals with particular psychiatric disorders often preferentially choose certain classes of substances. For example, patients with negative symptoms of Schizophrenia often prefer stimulants and patients with anxiety disorders often prefer CNS depressants. The hallmark of a primary psychiatric disorder with secondary substance use is that the primary psychiatric disorder occurs first and/or exists at times during the person's lifetime when he or she is not using any substance. In the most classic situation, the period of comorbid psychiatric symptomatology and substance use is immediately preceded by a period of time when the person had the psychiatric symptomatology but was abstinent from the substance. For example, an individual currently with 5 months of heavy alcohol use and depressive symptomatology might report that the alcohol use started in the midst of the depressive episode, perhaps as a way of counteracting the insomnia. Clearly the validity of this judgment depends on the accuracy of the patient's retrospective reporting. Because such information is sometimes suspect, it may be useful to confer with other informants (e.g., family members) or review past records to document the presence of psychiatric symptoms occurring in the absence of substance use.

Finally, both the psychiatric disorder and the substance use can be initially unrelated and independent of each other. The high prevalences of both psychiatric disorders and substance use disorders mean that, by chance alone, one would expect some patients to have two independent illnesses. Of course, however, even if initially independent, the two disorders may interact to exacerbate each other and complicate the overall treatment. This independent relationship is essentially a diagnosis made by exclusion. When confronted with a patient having both psychiatric symptomatology and substance use, you should first rule out that one is causing the other. A lack of a causal relationship in either direction is more likely if there are periods when the psychiatric symptoms occur in the absence of substance use and if the substance use occurs at times unrelated to the psychiatric symptomatology.

Once you have decided that a presentation is due to the direct effects of a substance, you must then determine which DSM-IV-TR Substance-Induced Disorder best describes the presentation. DSM-IV-TR includes a number of specific Substance-Induced Disorders, along with Substance Intoxication and Substance Withdrawal. Please refer to the "Decision Tree for Mental Disorder Due to Substance Use" in Chapter 2 (see p. 120) for a presentation of the steps involved in making this determination.

Step 3: Rule Out a Disorder Due to a General Medical Condition

After ruling out a substance-induced etiology, the next step is to determine whether the psychiatric symptoms are due to a general medical condition. This is one of the most important and difficult distinctions in psychiatric diagnosis. It is important because many individuals with general medical conditions have resulting psychiatric symptoms as a complication of the general medical condition and because many individuals with psychiatric symptoms have an underlying general medical condition. The treatment implications of this differential diagnostic step are also profound. Appropriate identification and treatment of the underlying general medical condition can be crucial in both avoiding medical complications and reducing the psychiatric symptomatology.

This differential diagnosis can be difficult for the following reasons: 1) symptoms of some psychiatric disorders and of many general medical conditions can be identical (e.g., symptoms of weight loss and fatigue can be attributable to a depressive or anxiety disorder or to a general medical condition), 2) sometimes the first presenting symptoms of a general medical condition are psychiatric (e.g., depression preceding other symptoms in pancreatic cancer, brain tumor), 3) the relationship between the general medical condition and the psychiatric symptoms may be complicated (e.g., depression or anxiety as a psychological reaction to having the medical condition versus the general medical condition being a cause of the depression or anxiety via its direct physiological effect on the CNS), and 4) patients are often seen in settings primarily geared for the identification and treatment of mental disorders in which there may be a lower expectation for, and familiarity with, the diagnosis of general medical conditions.

Virtually any psychiatric presentation can be caused by the direct physiological effects of a general medical condition, and these are diagnosed in DSM-IV-TR as one of the Mental Disorders Due to a General Medical Condition (e.g., Mood Disorder Due to Hypothyroidism). It is no great trick to suspect the possible etiological role of a general medical condition if the patient is encountered in a general hospital or primary care outpatient setting. The real diagnostic challenge occurs in mental health settings in which the base rate of general medical conditions is much lower but nonetheless consequential. It is not feasible (nor cost effective) to order every conceivable screening test on every patient. One should direct the history, physical examination, and laboratory tests toward the diagnosis of those general medical conditions that are most commonly encountered and most likely to account for the presenting psychiatric symptoms (e.g., thyroid function tests for depression, brain imaging for late-onset psychotic symptoms).

Once a general medical condition is established, the next step is to determine its etiological relationship, if any, to the psychiatric symptoms. The five possible relationships include 1) the general medical condition causes the psychiatric symptoms through a direct physiological effect on the brain,

2) the general medical condition causes the psychiatric symptoms through a psychological mechanism (e.g., depressive symptoms in response to being diagnosed with cancer—diagnosed as Major Depressive Disorder or Adjustment Disorder), 3) medication taken for the general medical condition causes the psychiatric symptoms (see "Step 2" in this chapter), 4) the psychiatric symptoms cause or adversely effect the general medical condition (e.g., in which case Psychological Factors Affecting Medical Condition may be indicated), and 5) the psychiatric symptoms and the general medical condition are coincidental (e.g., hypertension and Schizophrenia). In the real clinical world, however, several of these relationships may occur simultaneously with a multifactorial etiology (e.g., a patient treated with an antihypertensive medication who has a stroke may develop depression due to a combination of the direct effects of the stroke on the brain, the psychological reaction to the resultant paralysis, and as a side effect of the antihypertensive medication).

There are several clues suggesting that psychopathology is caused by the direct physiological effect of a general medical condition. Unfortunately, none of these is infallible, and clinical judgment is always necessary in their application.

The first clue involves the nature of the temporal relationship: Do the psychiatric symptoms begin following the onset of the general medical condition, vary in severity with the severity of the general medical condition, and disappear when the general medical condition resolves? When all of these relationships can be demonstrated, a fairly compelling case can be made that the general medical condition has caused the psychiatric symptoms, although it does not establish that the relationship is physiological (the temporal covariation could also be due to a psychological reaction to the general medical condition). Sometimes, however, the temporal relationship is not a good indicator of underlying etiology. For instance, psychiatric symptoms may be the first harbinger of the general medical condition and may precede by months or years any other manifestations. Conversely, psychiatric symptoms may be a relatively late manifestation occurring months or years after the general medical condition has been well established (e.g., depression in Parkinson's disease).

The second clue that a general medical condition should be considered in the differential diagnosis is if the psychiatric presentation is atypical in symptom pattern, age at onset, or course. For example, the presentation cries out for a medical workup when there is severe memory or weight loss accompanying a relatively mild depression or severe disorientation accompanying psychotic symptoms. Similarly, the first onset of a Manic Episode in an elderly patient may suggest that a general medical condition is involved in the etiology. However, atypicality does not in and of itself indicate a general medical etiology because the heterogeneity of primary disorders leads to many "atypical" presentations. Nonetheless, the most important bottom line with regard to this step in the differential diagnosis is not to miss possibly important underlying general medical conditions. Establishing the nature of the causal relationship often requires careful evaluation, longitudinal follow-up, and trials of treatment.

Finally, if you have determined that a general medical condition is responsible for the psychiatric symptoms, you must determine which of the DSM-IV-TR Mental Disorders Due to a General Medical Condition best describes the presentation. DSM-IV-TR includes a number of such disorders, each differentiated by the predominant symptom presentation. Please refer to the "Decision Tree for Mental Disorders Due to a General Medical Condition" in Chapter 2 (see p. 116) for a presentation of the steps involved in making this determination.

Step 4: Determine the Specific Primary Disorder(s)

Once substance use and general medical conditions have been ruled out as etiologies, your next task is to determine which among the primary DSM-IV-TR mental disorders best accounts for the presenting symptomatology. The sections of DSM-IV-TR are organized around common presenting symptoms (e.g., mood, anxiety, dissociative) precisely to facilitate this differential diagnosis. The decision trees in Chapter 2 provide the decision points needed for choosing among the primary mental disorders that might account for each symptom. Once you have selected what appears to be the most likely disorder, you may wish to review the pertinent differential diagnosis table in Chapter 3 to ensure that all other likely contenders in the differential diagnosis have been considered and ruled out.

Step 5: Differentiate Adjustment Disorder From Not Otherwise Specified

Many clinical presentations (particularly in outpatient and primary care settings) cause clinically significant distress or impairment but do not conform to the particular symptom patterns or fall below the established severity or duration thresholds to qualify for one of the specific DSM-IV-TR diagnoses. In such situations, a diagnosis of a mental disorder is warranted, and the differential comes down to either Adjustment Disorder or the appropriate Not Otherwise Specified category. If the clinical judgment is made that the symptoms have developed as a maladaptive response to a psychosocial stressor, the diagnosis would be Adjustment Disorder. If it is judged that a stressor is not responsible for the development of the symptoms, then the relevant Not Otherwise Specified category may be diagnosed. Because stress is a daily feature of most people's lives, the judgment in this step is centered more on whether a stressor is etiological rather than on whether a stressor is present.

Step 6: Establish the Boundary With No Mental Disorder

This is generally the last step in each of the decision trees but is by no means the least important or easiest to make. Taken individually, many of the symptoms included in DSM-IV-TR are fairly ubiquitous and are not by themselves indicative of the presence of a mental disorder. During the course of their lives, most people may experience periods of anxiety, depression, sleeplessness, or sexual dysfunction that may be considered as no more than an expected part of the human condition. To be explicit that not every such individual qualifies for a diagnosis of a mental disorder, DSM-IV added to most criteria sets an item that is usually worded more or less as follows: "The disturbance causes clinically significant distress or impairment in social, occupational, or other important areas of functioning." This requires that any psychopathology must lead to clinically significant problems in order to warrant a mental disorder diagnosis. For example, a diagnosis of Hypoactive Sexual Desire Disorder would not be made in someone with low sexual desire who is not currently in a relationship and who is not particularly bothered by it.

Unfortunately, but necessarily, DSM-IV-TR makes no attempt to define the term *clinically significant*. The boundary between disorder and normality can be set only by clinical judgment and not by any hard-and-fast rules. What may seem clinically significant is undoubtedly influenced by the cultural context, the setting in which the individual is seen, clinician bias, patient bias, and the availability of resources. "Minor" depression may seem much more clinically significant in a primary care setting than if it is seen in a psychiatric emergency room or state hospital where the emphasis is on the identification and treatment of far more impairing conditions. This is a very controversial area of great public health significance and relevance to treatment decisions and benefit entitlements. It will require considerable additional research in order to inform policy decisions.

Differential Diagnosis and Comorbidity

Differential diagnosis is generally based on the notion that one is choosing a single diagnosis from among a group of competing mutually exclusive diagnoses to best explain a given symptom presentation. For example, in a patient who presents with delusions, hallucinations, and mood symptoms, the question is whether the best diagnosis is Schizophrenia, Schizoaffective Disorder, or Mood Disorder With Psychotic Features—only one of these can be given to describe the current presentation. Very often, however, DSM-IV-TR diagnoses are not mutually exclusive, and the assignment of more than one DSM-IV-TR diagnosis to a given patient is both allowed and necessary to adequately describe the presenting symptoms. For example, there is no single DSM-IV-TR diagnosis that describes a commonly encountered patient who presents with multiple unexpected panic attacks, significant depression, and a maladaptively perfectionistic and rigid personality style. Instead, three DSM-IV-TR diagnoses are needed for this presentation: Major Depressive Disorder, Panic Disorder, and Obsessive-Compulsive Personality Disorder. In this instance, it is not a question of choosing one "best" diagnosis but rather indicating which diagnoses apply.

It is important that the reader understand that the decision trees in Chapter 2 and the symptom index in Chapter 4 present the diagnoses that might apply to a given symptom without indicating which of these are mutually exclusive. To have done so would have rendered the trees and the index impossibly complicated to use. Instead, the information regarding which diagnoses cannot be given together is contained in the differential diagnosis tables in Chapter 3. For example, in Chapter 2, the "Decision Tree for Physical Complaints or Irrational Anxiety About Apperance" does not provide the rules governing the relationships among Somatization Disorder,

Conversion Disorder, and Pain Disorder. By just reviewing the tree, there is no way that one would know that the DSM-IV-TR criteria prevent the diagnosis of Conversion Disorder and Pain Disorder if criteria are met for the more pervasive diagnosis of Somatization Disorder (which includes conversion and pain symptoms). Furthermore, the tree does not tell you that in the absence of Somatization Disorder a diagnosis of Conversion Disorder is compatible with a comorbid diagnosis of Pain Disorder if a patient has both pain and conversion symptoms. A look at the differential diagnosis tables for Somatization Disorder, Conversion Disorder, and Pain Disorder in Chapter 3 clarifies these relationships.

The use of multiple diagnoses is in itself neither good nor bad so long as the implications are understood. A naive and mistaken view of comorbidity might assume that a patient assigned more than one descriptive diagnosis actually has multiple independent conditions. This is certainly not the only possible relationship. In fact, there are six different ways in which two "comorbid conditions" may be related to one another: 1) condition A may cause or predispose to condition B, 2) condition B may cause or predispose to condition A, 3) an underlying condition C may cause or predispose to both conditions A and B, 4) conditions A and B may in fact be part of a more complex unified syndrome that has been artificially split in the diagnostic system, 5) the relationship between conditions A and B may be artifactually enhanced by definitional overlap, and 6) the comorbidity is the result of a chance co-occurrence that may be particularly likely for those conditions that have high base rates. The particular nature of the relationships is often very difficult to determine. The major point to keep in mind is that "having" more than one DSM-IV-TR diagnosis does not mean that there is more than one underlying pathophysiological process. Instead, DSM-IV-TR diagnoses should be considered descriptive building blocks that are useful for communicating diagnostic information.

How to Use the Handbook: A Case Example

Perhaps a brief case illustration will demonstrate how this handbook can be used to facilitate differential diagnosis. One of the most common and complicated differential diagnoses encountered in clinical practice involves a patient who presents with depressive symptoms and evidence of substance use. Probably the best starting point would be to refer to the "Decision Tree for Depressed Mood" in Chapter 2 (see p. 46). Almost immediately, you are advised to consider the possible etiological role of the substance use in causing the depressive symptoms. Your next step would be to refer back to this chapter for a detailed discussion of how best to determine whether the depression is a direct result of the substance use, whether the substance use is a form of self-medication for the preexisting depression, or whether they are independent. Let's say that you determine that the depressive symptoms are not due to either a substance or a general medical condition. You would then continue through the tree to determine which particular DSM-IV-TR disorder best accounts for the depressed mood. Once you have arrived at a tentative decision (e.g., Major Depressive Disorder), you might then refer to the differential diagnosis table for Major Depressive Disorder in Chapter 3 (see p. 154) to double-check that all other contenders have been considered and ruled out. In Chapter 4, the symptom index entry for depressed mood (see p. 221) provides a quicker alternative to the decision trees if one is interested in learning which disorders should be considered in the differential diagnosis.

Differential Diagnosis by the Trees

D ecision trees are a convenient means of elucidating the steps that inform differential diagnosis. Each decision tree starts with a particular presenting symptom and then provides decision points for determining which diagnosis may best account for it. For any given patient, several trees may (and often do) apply. In many instances, following the branches within the different pertinent decision trees will lead to the same diagnosis, suggesting that the presenting symptoms constitute a single syndrome. In other instances, more than one diagnosis may be indicated.

The first step in using these decision trees is to determine which ones apply to the clinical presentation. The presenting symptom for each tree is listed in the shaded box in the upper left. The yellow boxes (i.e., diagnostic endpoints) indicate all of the disorders that need to be considered in the differential diagnosis of the particular symptom. Intermediate boxes indicate how different disorders are ruled in or ruled out.

The reader should remember that the decision trees are no more than an overview of the diagnostic system and a guide to differential diagnosis. They should not be applied in a cookbook fashion. The decision trees contain only abbreviated versions of the diagnostic criteria and are simplified so that the disorders appear to be mutually exclusive. In fact, this is usually not the case; DSM-IV-TR encourages multiple diagnoses when criteria are met for more than one disorder. Therefore, the full criteria sets for the disorders should be referred to when making a diagnosis and determining whether multiple diagnoses are allowed. Referring to the pertinent differential diagnosis tables in Chapter 3 may also be helpful in this regard.

Many of the decision trees follow a standard format that mirrors the stepwise thought process used in making a differential diagnosis. The first consideration is whether the particular symptom is the result of the direct effects of a general medical condition or substance use. The next steps in the decision tree typically cover the primary mental disorders that may account for the symptom. The final step in most of the decision trees covers those presentations that do not conform to or fall below the threshold for a specific DSM-IV-TR diagnosis and may best be considered as an Adjustment Disorder, a Not Otherwise Specified disorder, or no mental disorder. The important step of determining whether the presenting symptom has been feigned (as in Malingering or Factitious Disorder) has generally not been included in the decision trees because it applies to the evaluation of all presenting symptoms.

The decision trees are presented in two sections. The first section is based on the presenting symptom and includes 24 decision trees. The second section is based on the presumed etiology and includes three trees: one for presentations that are due to a general medical condition, one for substance-induced presentations, and one for presentations related to a psychosocial stressor. This section is most useful in situations where the etiology is established (e.g., the patient has chronic substance use), but the specific disorder needs to be determined.

Trees Based on Presenting Symptoms

Decision Tree for Aggressive Behavior

Although aggressive behavior is a complication of a number of mental disorders, the psychiatric nosology of aggression has not been well worked out. Perhaps even more important to note is that most violent behavior occurs for reasons very far afield from the domain of mental illness (e.g., for material gain, status, sadistic pleasure, revenge, to further a political or religious cause). Moreover, even when the aggressive behavior is associated with a mental disorder, this fact does not by itself absolve the individual of criminal responsibility.

Among the DSM-IV-TR disorders, the Substance Use Disorders are by far the most frequent cause of aggressive behavior. Although the association is much less prominent, recent evidence also suggests that episodes of aggressive behavior may occur at somewhat elevated rates in individuals with Schizophrenia, Bipolar Disorder, and other psychotic disorders. A longstanding pattern of aggressive behavior suggests that the behavior is part of a Personality Disorder (or Conduct Disorder). Aggression can also result from the cognitive impairment and reduction in impulse control that is characteristic of Dementia and Delirium. When the aggressive behavior is a direct physiological consequence of a general medical condition but occurs in the absence of cognitive impairment, Personality Change Due to a General Medical Condition should be diagnosed. One issue that sometimes arises in the diagnosis of Personality Change Due to a General Medical Condition is whether to consider nonspecific medical findings (e.g., neurological soft signs, diffuse slowing on EEG) as evidence of a causative general medical condition. The DSM-IV-TR convention is to diagnose Personality Change only if the findings constitute a diagnosable general medical condition that would be coded on Axis III. However, the general medical code 348.9, Unspecified Condition of Brain, can be specified as the causative disorder and coded on Axis III when clinical judgment strongly suggests that a CNS dysfunction is present and responsible for the personality change but no specific diagnosis can be made. Patterns of aggressive behavior that are not attributable to a recurrent Axis I Disorder or to a Personality Disorder may qualify for a diagnosis of Intermittent Explosive Disorder.

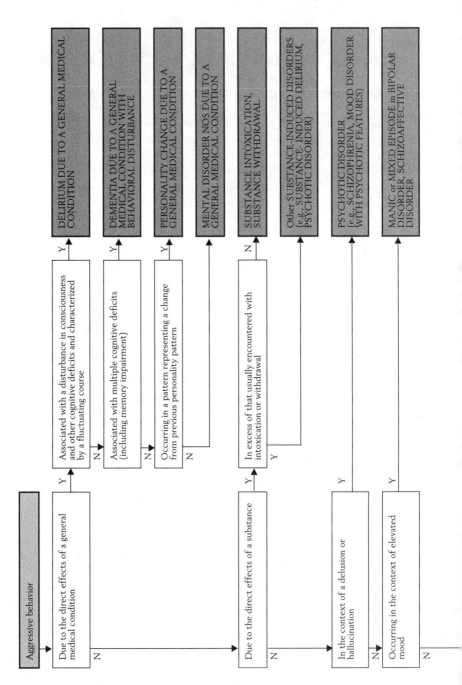

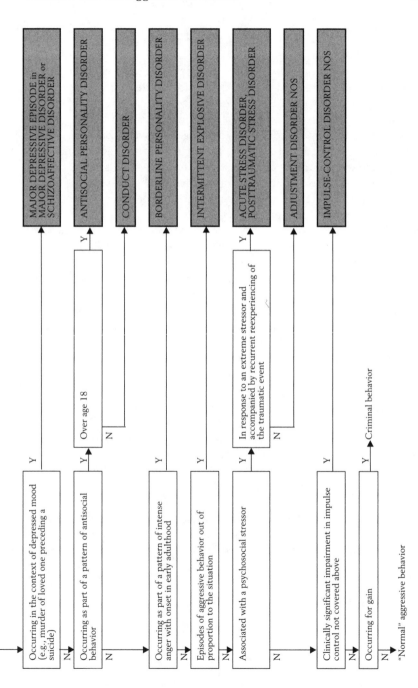

Decision Tree for Anxiety

As is always the case, the first step in the differential diagnosis is to rule out a general medical condition or substance use as the direct physiological cause of the anxiety. When the anxiety occurs in discrete episodes with a sudden onset and is accompanied by a number of somatic (e.g., palpitations, shortness of breath, dizziness) and cognitive symptoms (e.g., fear of going crazy or having a heart attack), it is diagnosed as a "panic attack." Because of the specific treatment implications of panic attacks, a separate decision tree is also provided for them (see Chapter 3 of this book).

The remaining differential steps in this tree are determined by the content of the anxiety. It is important in the assessment to determine what the individual is afraid of, the situations that are avoided, and whether the anxiety is in response to a stressor. In Panic Disorder, With or Without Agoraphobia, the anxiety is related to the fear of having additional panic attacks and the possible consequences of these attacks. Agoraphobia Without History of Panic Disorder is similar except that the individual has never had full-blown panic attacks and instead is afraid of having panic-like symptoms that are subthreshold to a panic attack (e.g., fainting, loss of bowel control). Separation Anxiety Disorder, Social Phobia, Specific Phobia, and Obsessive-Compulsive Disorder are related, respectively, to fears of being separated from an attachment figure, fears of social humiliation, fears of exposure to circumscribed objects or situations (e.g., heights, blood, elevators, spiders), and fears of triggering obsessive ruminations (e.g., of contamination, hurting someone). In Hypochondriasis and Body Dysmorphic Disorder, the anxiety is related to concerns about having a serious illness or bodily defect. Generalized Anxiety Disorder is a residual category for chronic anxiety and worry that is difficult to control. In contrast to Panic Disorder, the anxiety in this condition does not have a crescendo, attack-like quality with a sharp onset or offset.

The tree concludes with three disorders describing anxiety that occurs in response to a stressor. Two of these (Acute Stress Disorder and Posttraumatic Stress Disorder) require a stressor of a life- or limb-threatening nature, whereas for Adjustment Disorder, the stressor can be of a lesser severity.

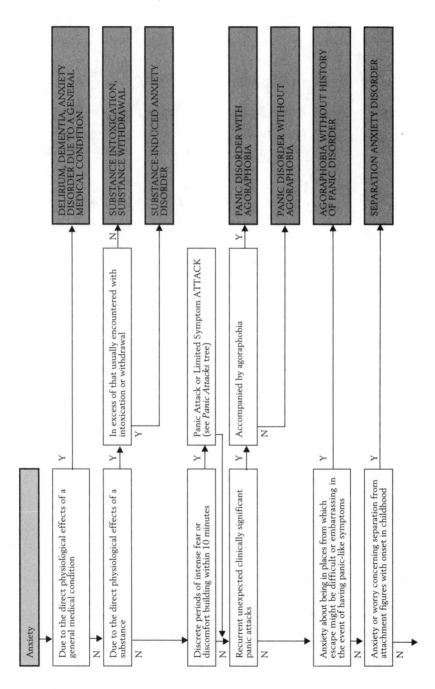

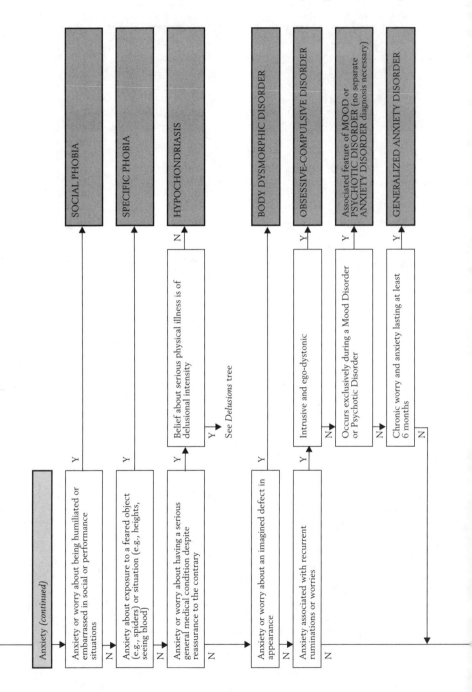

Anxiety *(continued)*

Anxiety or worry about being humiliated or embarrassed in social or performance situations — Y → **SOCIAL PHOBIA**

N ↓

Anxiety about exposure to a feared object (e.g., spiders) or situation (e.g., heights, seeing blood) — Y → **SPECIFIC PHOBIA**

N ↓

Anxiety or worry about having a serious general medical condition despite reassurance to the contrary — Y → Belief about serious physical illness is of delusional intensity — N → **HYPOCHONDRIASIS**

Y ↓

See *Delusions* tree

N ↓

Anxiety or worry about an imagined defect in appearance — Y → **BODY DYSMORPHIC DISORDER**

N ↓

Anxiety associated with recurrent ruminations or worries — Y → Intrusive and ego-dystonic — Y → **OBSESSIVE-COMPULSIVE DISORDER**

N ↓

Occurs exclusively during a Mood Disorder or Psychotic Disorder — Y → Associated feature of MOOD or PSYCHOTIC DISORDER (no separate ANXIETY DISORDER diagnosis necessary)

N ↓

Chronic worry and anxiety lasting at least 6 months — Y → **GENERALIZED ANXIETY DISORDER**

N ↓

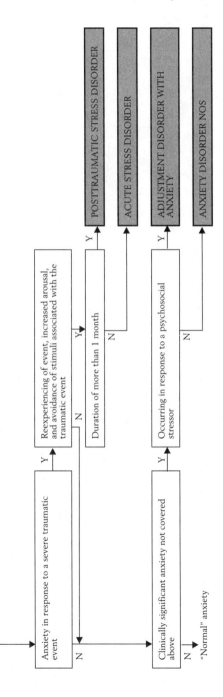

Decision Tree for Avoidance Behavior

Avoidance behavior (particularly of realistically harmful situations) is often adaptive. This decision tree applies only when the avoidance is based on unrealistic fears and leads to significant distress or impairment. Avoidance is a fairly ubiquitous and nonspecific symptom and is an associated feature of many disorders. The evaluation of this symptom requires determining the specific circumstances triggering the avoidance. The first order of business is determining whether the person has had panic attacks or panic-like symptoms and, if so, whether the panic attacks or symptoms are the cause of the avoidance—in which case the diagnosis is Panic Disorder With Agoraphobia (for panic attacks) or Agoraphobia Without History of Panic Disorder (for panic-like symptoms). Individuals associate the risk of having a panic attack with particular locations or situations that then become conditioned stimuli particularly likely to trigger additional attacks. They then avoid such "triggering" situations in an effort to minimize the chance of having panic attacks or panic-like symptoms.

The avoidance in Social Phobia is related to fear of social embarrassment. This avoidance comes in two forms (although some individuals are intermediate). The performance anxiety form of Social Phobia concerns avoidance of public activities (e.g., speaking, playing music, acting, eating, urinating, writing) that can easily be performed by the individual in the privacy of his or her own home. The generalized form includes virtually any situation that involves social interaction and in many cases may be virtually identical to Avoidant Personality Disorder. The Specific Phobias probably involve some interaction between evolutionarily predetermined, inborn fears and the occurrence of aversive early life experiences that reinforce them. Some individuals with Obsessive-Compulsive Disorder learn that avoiding certain triggering situations will prevent the onset of obsessions (e.g., avoidance of handshakes will help reduce contamination obsessions). In Posttraumatic Stress Disorder and Acute Stress Disorder, the individual avoids situations that are reminiscent of the stressor in any way (e.g., someone who resembles the assailant, loud sounds that recall wartime, tremors that recall a major earthquake). Many other psychiatric disorders can have avoidance as an associated feature (e.g., a delusional patient who avoids going outside for fear that the FBI is after him or her).

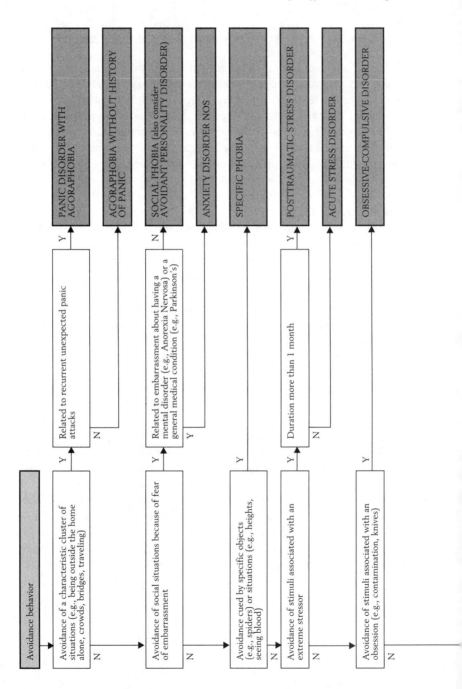

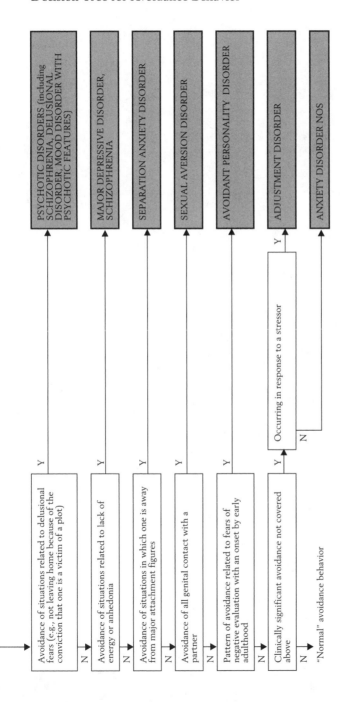

Decision Tree for Behavior Problems in a Child or Adolescent

A common reason for referring a child or adolescent to a mental health professional is to request an evaluation and possible treatment for a "behavior problem." It goes without saying, however, that many behavior problems occurring in children or adolescents are not due to a mental disorder. In some instances, the behaviors are not of sufficient severity or duration to warrant such a diagnosis. In others, the disturbance is more in the family relationship rather than in a problem emanating primarily from the child. Finally, there are some very serious behavior problems (e.g., shooting, mugging, rape) that occur for reasons outside the domain of the mental disorders covered in DSM-IV-TR (e.g., financial gain, status, revenge).

Behavior problems with an onset in infancy or early childhood are most often associated with Attention-Deficit/Hyperactivity Disorder, Pervasive Developmental Disorder, Mental Retardation, and Stereotyped Movement Disorder. The differential among these is usually straightforward and is determined by a consideration of the accompanying symptoms.

A first onset of behavior problems during adolescence strongly suggests that substances may play an important role. The behavior problems may result from the direct effect of the substance on the brain (as in Substance Intoxication), may be a by-product of a Substance Dependence or Abuse (e.g., illegal activities associated with procurement), or may be motivated by gain (e.g., getting rich quick as a drug dealer). Other disorders that can be associated with an adolescent onset include a better prognosis form of Conduct Disorder, Major Depressive Disorder, Bipolar Disorder, and Schizophrenia. Conduct Disorder can also have an onset in childhood (i.e., prior to age 10). This form of Conduct Disorder is particularly worrisome and is associated with a higher incidence of violence, poorer peer relationships, and an increased likelihood for the child to develop into an adult with Antisocial Personality Disorder.

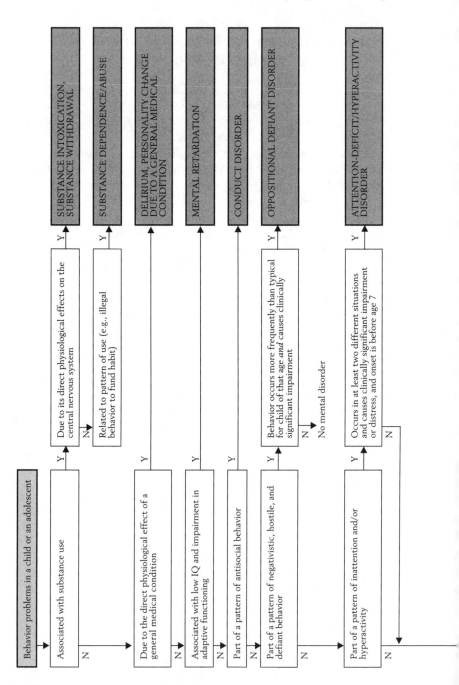

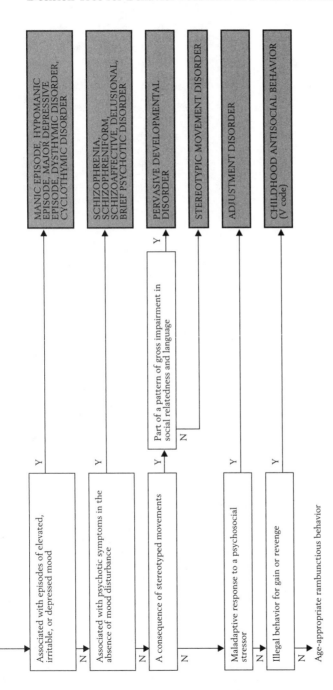

Decision Tree for Catatonia

The catatonic symptoms covered here include motoric immobility (waxy flexibility or stupor), catatonic excitement (excessive purposeless motor activity), extreme negativism or catatonic mutism, catatonic posturing or stereotypies, or echolalia or echopraxia. DSM-IV (and DSM-IV-TR) should help to correct a common error in regard to the differential diagnosis of Catatonia. Most clinicians tend to associate Catatonia exclusively with Schizophrenia despite the fact that most instances of Catatonia occur instead in association with mood episodes, neurological conditions, or medication side effects. DSM-IV highlighted and expanded the differential diagnosis of catatonic symptoms by adding the With Catatonic Features specifier for Mood Disorders, by including a new section for Medication-Induced Movement Disorders, and by introducing a new disorder, Catatonic Disorder Due to a General Medical Condition.

The initial task is to determine whether a catatonic "syndrome" is present. This can be difficult because a number of the individual items resemble other types of symptoms characteristic of DSM-IV-TR disorders (e.g., catatonic excitement may resemble psychomotor agitation in a Manic or Major Depressive Episode, catatonic stupor may resemble extreme psychomotor retardation in a Major Depressive Episode or delirium, catatonic mutism may resemble alogia and avolition in Schizophrenia). The judgment about these distinctions is based in part on the context in which the symptom occurs (i.e., the presence of multiple catatonic symptoms vs. the presence of symptoms characteristic of the other disorder) and on its presentation (i.e., individuals with catatonic symptoms appear to be oblivious to external environmental stimuli although they may later report accurately about what was happening around them).

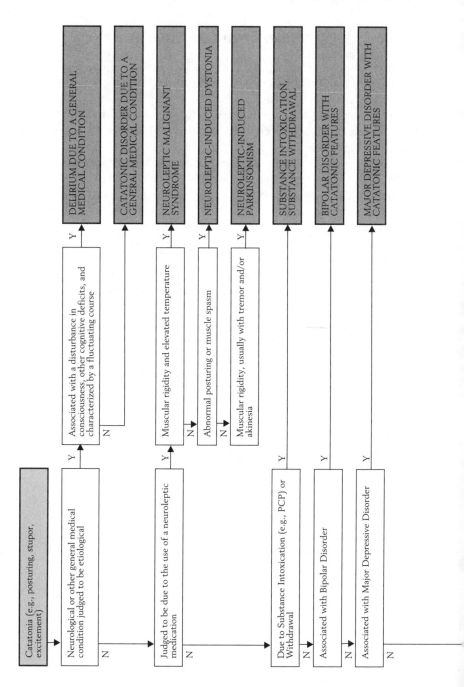

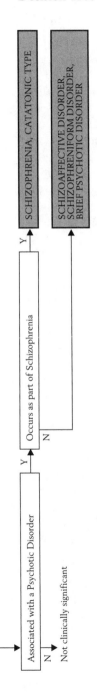

Associated with a Psychotic Disorder

Y → Occurs as part of Schizophrenia

Y → SCHIZOPHRENIA, CATATONIC TYPE

N → SCHIZOAFFECTIVE DISORDER, SCHIZOPHRENIFORM DISORDER, BRIEF PSYCHOTIC DISORDER

N → Not clinically significant

Decision Tree for Changes in Appetite or Unusual Eating Behavior

This decision tree covers several disparate symptoms associated with eating: weight and appetite changes, binge eating, rumination, and pica. Because changes in appetite and weight are commonly caused by general medical conditions, your first thought should always be to rule out cancer, endocrine disturbances, chronic infections, and other illnesses before assuming that the symptoms are psychiatric. This is especially the case when weight loss or gain is of major proportions and occurs in conjunction with other physical symptoms. Moreover, changes in appetite and weight (in both directions) are also frequently caused by the use of certain drugs of abuse (especially stimulants and cannabis) and certain prescribed medications. In fact, one of the major reasons for noncompliance with many of the psychotropic medications (e.g., tricyclic antidepressants, lithium, monoamine oxidase inhibitors, neuroleptics) is the fear of weight gain that commonly accompanies their use. Attributing changes in weight can be difficult precisely because many of the conditions treated by these psychotropics are themselves associated with changes in weight independent of the use of medication. For example, if a depressed patient gains weight while being treated with an antidepressant, this could be a side effect of the antidepressant, a characteristic symptom of the depression, or a desirable treatment effect (e.g., improved appetite in someone previously experiencing loss of appetite).

Because changes in appetite and gains or losses in weight are so common in so many different psychiatric disorders, they are relatively nonspecific in providing clues to the differential diagnosis. Therefore, you must rely on the pattern of, and temporal relationship with, the other presenting symptoms in deciding which is the most appropriate explanation for the change in appetite or weight. For example, is the individual not eating because of a delusion that the food is poisoned (as in Delusional Disorder), because of a feeling of being unworthy or a loss of pleasure in eating (as in Major Depressive Episode), or as a result of a diminished appetite or being "too busy" (as in Manic Episode)?

In some individuals, weight loss or weight gain is associated with a specific presentation of severe body image distortions and/or binge eating. DSM-IV-TR includes a separate section for Eating Disorders (Anorexia Nervosa, Bulimia Nervosa) that are characterized by special eating behaviors associated with overemphasis on body image. In Anorexia Nervosa, the pathological fear of being (or becoming) fat results in an often dangerously low weight. Some individuals with Anorexia Nervosa engage in binge eating and purging behavior, whereas others achieve low weight exclusively through fasting and excessive exercise. In contrast to those with Anorexia Nervosa, individuals with Bulimia Nervosa have normal or above normal weight. They engage in cycles of binge eating compensated for by the use of inappropriate methods of counteracting the effects of their excessive caloric intake (e.g., self-induced vomiting, misuse of laxatives, fasting, excessive exercise).

The decision tree also contains several eating disturbances that occur primarily in infants, young children, or individuals with Mental Retardation. Pica is the developmentally inappropriate and persistent eating of nonnutritive substances (e.g., paint chips, string, dirt, animal droppings). Rumination Disorder is the repeated regurgitation and rechewing of food. Feeding Disorder of Infancy or Early Childhood is a residual category for severe weight loss (or failure of weight gain) that usually results from a combination of a difficult-to-feed child and an inexperienced caretaker.

Finally, it is important to remember that concern about body appearance, gaining and losing weight, and fad dieting are fairly ubiquitous aspects of life in the developed world and usual do not by themselves warrant a diagnosis of a mental disorder. Moreover, it should be noted that obesity is not considered a mental disorder because it is not yet clear the degree to which psychological factors play a role in its pathogenesis.

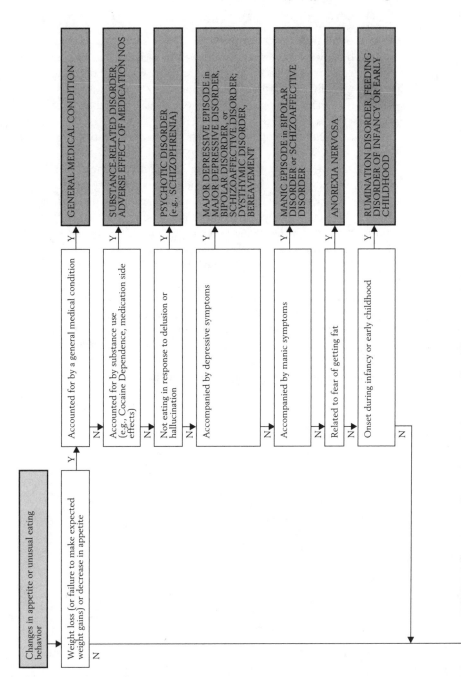

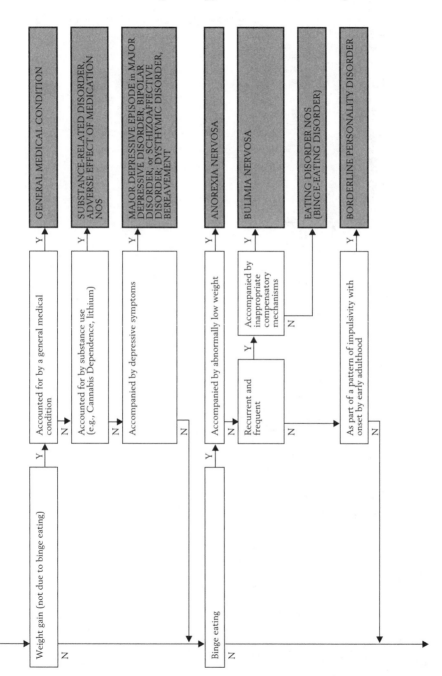

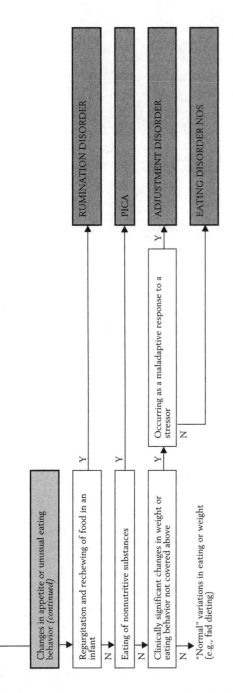

Decision Tree for Delusions

A common error regarding the differential diagnosis in this decision tree is to assume that a belief that is unusual (at least from the clinician's perspective) is necessarily a delusion. Such misattributions can be avoided through a careful application of the DSM-IV-TR glossary definition of delusion:

> A false belief based on incorrect inference about external reality that is firmly sustained despite what almost everyone else believes and despite what constitutes incontrovertible and obvious proof or evidence to the contrary. The belief is not one ordinarily accepted by other members of the person's culture or subculture (e.g., it is not an article of religious faith). When a false belief involves a value judgment, it is regarded as a delusion only when the judgment is so extreme as to defy credibility. Delusional conviction occurs on a continuum and can be sometimes be inferred from an individual's behavior. It is often difficult to distinguish between a delusion and an overvalued idea (in which case the individual has an unreasonable belief or idea but does not hold it as firmly as is the case with a delusion).

Several aspects of this definition are helpful to keep in mind when attempting to determine whether a patient is delusional. Delusional convictions are impervious to compelling evidence of their implausibility, and the person remains totally convinced of their voracity, rejecting alternative explanations out of hand. In deciding whether a belief is fixed and false enough to be considered a delusion, you must first determine that a serious error in inference and reality testing has occurred and then determine the strength of the conviction. It may be helpful to ask the patient to talk at length about his or her conviction because it is often only in the specific details that the errors of inference become apparent. In evaluating the strength of the delusional conviction, you should present alternative explanations (e.g., the possibility that the phone hang-ups are due to people dialing a wrong number). The patient who cannot even acknowledge the possibility of these explanations is most likely to be delusional. When you are unfamiliar with the beliefs characteristic of the individual's cultural or religious background, consultation with another individual who is familiar with the patient's culture may be required to avoid the overdiagnosis of delusions. In our experience, the more common error is the overdiagnosis rather than the underdiagnosis of the presence of delusions, and in uncertain cases you should probably give the patient the benefit of the doubt.

Once it is determined that a delusion is present, your next task is to determine which from among the many possible DSM-IV-TR disorders best accounts for it. The particular content and form of a delusion are much less important in making the diagnosis than is the context in which it occurs. The most common diagnostic error here is to overlook the critically important role of substances (including medications) and general medical conditions in the etiology of delusions. In younger individuals presenting with delusions, it is important to do a careful history and drug screening to rule out the role of drugs of abuse. A late first onset of delusional thinking should always raise a red flag for a possible underlying general medical condition or medication side effect.

Once a general medical and substance etiology has been ruled out, the next task is to determine whether clinically significant mood symptoms are also present. The presence of a Major Depressive, Manic, or Mixed Episode raises the possibility that the delusions are part of a Mood Disorder With Psychotic Features or Schizoaffective Disorder. The differential diagnosis here depends on the timing of the delusions and the mood symptoms. If delusions are confined exclusively to the mood episode, then the diagnosis is a Mood Disorder With Psychotic Features. On the other hand, if delusions and other psychotic symptoms also occur before or after the mood episode, the diagnosis might be either Schizophrenia, Delusional Disorder, or Schizoaffective Disorder, depending on the relative significance of the mood versus the psychotic symptoms. The diagnosis is Schizophrenia or Delusional Disorder if the mood symptoms are only a brief part of the total psychotic disturbance (e.g., several months of mood during a chronic psychotic disturbance). In contrast, the diagnosis is Schizoaffective Disorder if the mood episodes constitute a significant part of the clinical picture (e.g., a 2-year psychotic disturbance with a year of mood symptoms).

Once you have ruled out significant mood episodes, the differential diagnosis depends on symptom pattern and duration. The distinction between Schizophrenia and Delusional Disorder is usually based on the presence in Schizophrenia of one or more additional symptoms (e.g., hallucinations, disorganized speech, disorganized behavior, negative symptoms). Occasionally, however, the diagnostic boundary between Schizophrenia and Delusional Disorder depends solely on the content of the delusion—a bizarre content rules out Delusional Disorder.

The duration of the episode is what distinguishes Schizophrenia, Schizophreniform Disorder, and Brief Psychotic Disorder. A duration of 1 month or less would be diagnosed as Brief Psychotic Disorder; 1–6 months' duration would be Schizophreniform Disorder, and over 6 months' duration would be Schizophrenia.

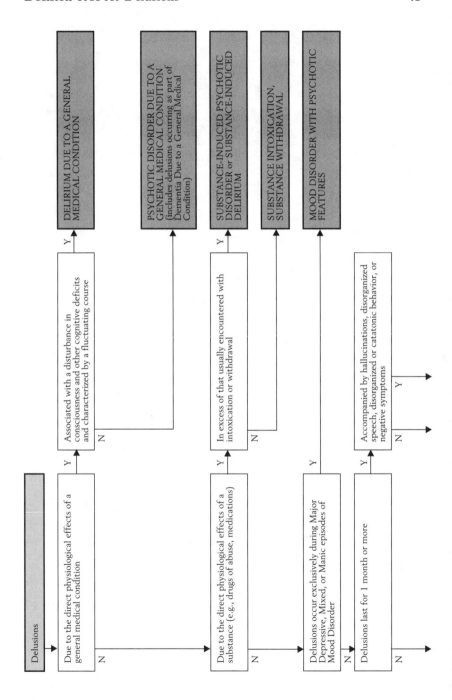

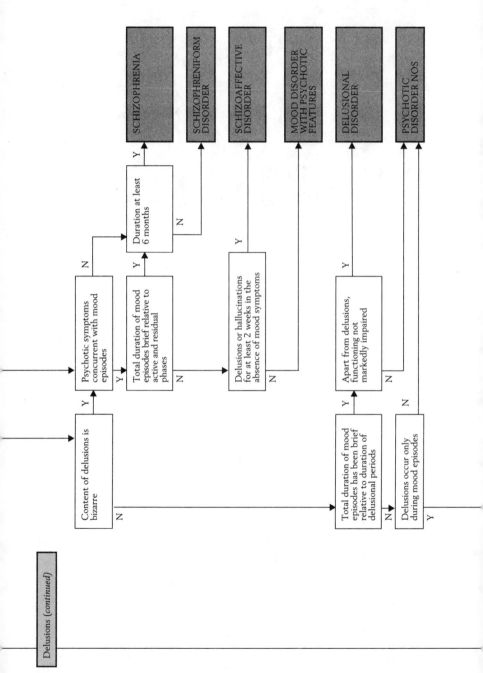

Delusions (*continued*)

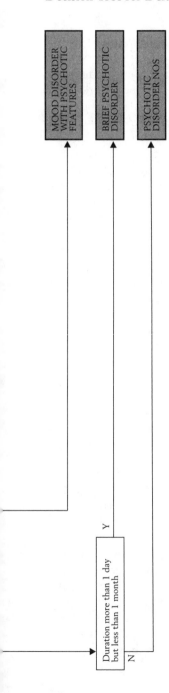

Decision Tree for Depressed Mood

Depressed or dysphoric mood is one of the most common presenting symptoms in mental health settings and is a component of many psychiatric conditions. It is important to consider the context in which the depression occurs and the clustering and duration of symptoms. One of the most difficult differential diagnostic determinations in psychiatry is to distinguish between primary mood disorders and those that are the direct physiological consequences of a general medical condition. A very large number of general medical conditions are known to cause depression through their direct effect on the brain. If severe cognitive impairment is also present, Dementia along with a Mood Disorder Due to a General Medical Condition must be considered. However, it is important not to assume that the severity of the cognitive impairment necessarily indicates a diagnosis of Dementia. The cognitive impairment that occurs as part of a Major Depressive Episode can be so severe as to mimic a dementia. Often, only time, serial evaluations, and sequential treatment trials will confirm whether a particular presentation is better explained by a Dementia along with a Mood Disorder Due to a General Medical Condition or a Major Depressive Episode with severe cognitive symptoms.

Substances (including both drugs of abuse and medication side effects) must also be ruled out. Depression can arise either during intoxication with certain substances (e.g., cannabis) or else be part of the withdrawal (e.g., cocaine). Because depressed mood is a frequent concomitant of intoxication and withdrawal, it usually does not require a separate diagnosis. However, if the depressed mood is a focus of clinical attention and is in excess of that usually encountered with intoxication or withdrawal, a diagnosis of Substance-Induced Mood Disorder may be appropriate. The differential between Substance-Induced Mood Disorder and primary Mood Disorder can be made historically by documenting that the depressed mood occurs only in relation to substance use. When such a history is not forthcoming, a period of abstinence is usually required to determine whether the depressed mood resolves once the effects of the substance wear off. DSM-IV-TR suggests waiting "about a month" after cessation of substance use to see whether the mood symptoms spontaneously resolve, although the actual time frame varies depending on the drug and the clinical situation. Other factors that should be considered include previous history of primary mood episodes, family history, and whether the depression is characteristic of the substance. If the mood symptoms persist after a reasonable waiting period, then a Substance-Induced Disorder is unlikely and the diagnosis is a primary Mood Disorder.

The next step of the differential diagnosis is to determine whether the depressed mood is part of a Mood Episode (e.g., Major Depressive Episode or Mixed Episode). These episodes are not coded separately in DSM-IV-TR but form the building blocks for the Mood Disorders (e.g., Major Depressive Disorder, Bipolar I Disorder). A Major Depressive Episode requires a minimum duration of at least 2 weeks of depressed mood for most of the day, nearly every day. Furthermore, the depressed mood must be accompanied by at least four additional symptoms over the same time period (e.g., changes in appetite or weight, sleep, level of motor activity, and suicidal ideation). If the criteria are simultaneously met for a Manic Episode, then the combination of depressive and manic symptoms is considered in DSM-IV-TR to be a Mixed Episode.

Because of its important treatment implications, the main conceptual division in the Mood Disorders section of DSM-IV-TR is between "unipolar" disorders and "bipolar" disorders. The next three steps in the decision tree serve to identify those individuals whose current presentation is depressed but whose overall course is characteristic of one of the Bipolar Disorders. Depressive symptoms accompanied by a history of Manic Episodes indicate Bipolar I Disorder, Hypomanic Episodes with Major Depressive Episodes indicate Bipolar II Disorder, and chronic depressive symptoms alternating with hypomanic periods warrant a diagnosis of Cyclothymic Disorder.

For unipolar depressive presentations, the specific diagnosis depends on the presence of Major Depressive Episodes, in which case the diagnosis is either Major Depressive Disorder or Schizoaffective Disorder (e.g., psychotic symptoms persist in the absence of prominent depression). Dysthymic Disorder is characterized by chronic depression that is below the symptom threshold for a Major Depressive Episode.

Depending on the circumstances, depressed mood that occurs in response to a stressor can be characteristic of several different disorders. If the stressor is the death of loved one, Bereavement (not a mental disorder) should be considered. If the depressive symptoms are particularly severe or prolonged, then a diagnosis of Major Depressive Disorder may be more appropriate even if the depression occurs after the loss of a loved one. For other stressors (e.g., loss of job), if the depressive reaction meets the full criteria for a specific Mood Disorder (e.g., Major Depressive Disorder), then that diagnosis is made. Maladaptive reactions that include depressive symptoms but do not meet the criteria for a specific Mood Disorder are classifiable as Adjustment Disorder With Depressed Mood.

It should be noted that the presence of depressed mood does not neces-sarily imply a diagnosis of a mood disorder. Many DSM-IV-TR disorders are accompanied by depressive symptoms, often as a form of "demoralization." In such cases, the separate mood disorder diagnosis (Depressive Disorder NOS) is justified only if the depressive symptoms are particularly severe and require independent clinical attention. Furthermore, the "blues" are a normal part of everyday life and do not warrant a diagnosis unless they lead to clinically significant distress or impairment.

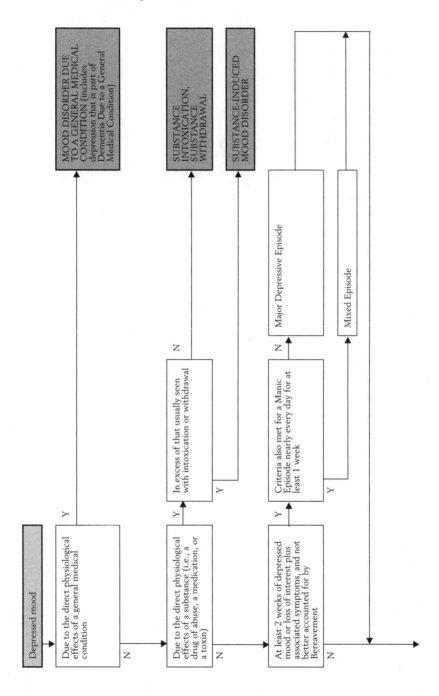

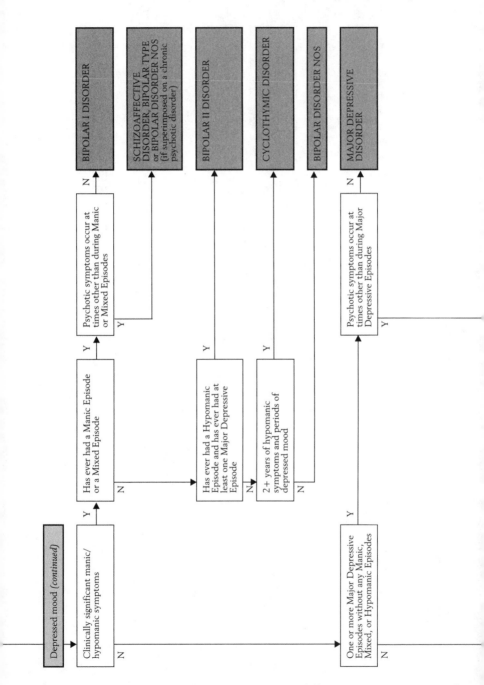

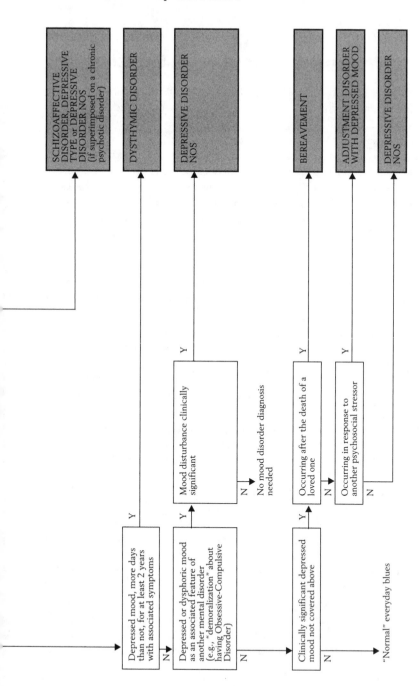

Decision Tree for
Disorganized or Unusual Speech

This is one of the most challenging symptoms to diagnose because there is no standard by which to judge when speech is "disorganized." This judgment depends in part on your ability to comprehend as well as the patient's pattern of speech production. Furthermore, no one speaks in logically coherent and syntactically correct sentences all the time. Our experience suggests that many clinicians and trainees have a tendency to overcall mildly illogical speech as clinically significant "loosening of associations." The kinds of "disorganized" or "unusual" speech covered in this decision tree should be obvious even to the most casual observer. If you have difficulty deciding whether or not a patient's speech is disorganized, then it should probably not be considered pathological.

Once it is established that there is disorganized or unusual speech, the next challenge is to determine which of the many possible mental disorders best accounts for it. This usually requires an evaluation of the context and the accompanying symptoms. Speech disturbance that is due to a general medical condition may be diagnosed as aphasia, Delirium, or Dementia depending on which other symptoms are present. The speech disturbance in Delirium is accompanied by a clouding in consciousness; in Dementia it is accompanied by clinically significant memory impairment. Aphasia (defined in DSM-IV-TR as an "impairment in the understanding or transmission of ideas by language . . . due to injury or disease of the brain centers involved in language") that occurs in the absence of other cognitive symptoms can be diagnosed by using the ICD-9-CM symptom code 784.3.

Disorganized speech is a common manifestation of substance use. Usually a diagnosis of Substance Intoxication or Withdrawal will suffice, but severely disorganized speech suggests a diagnosis of Substance-Induced Delirium or an underlying Substance-Induced Persisting Dementia.

The differential diagnosis of disorganized speech in mania vs. Schizophrenia has been the subject of considerable discussion. The disorganized speech in an episode of Schizophrenia (e.g., so-called loosening of associations) presumably is distinguished from the "flight of ideas" in mania based on the observer's ability to follow the train of thought. Theoretically, at least, one can discern how the patient got from one topic to the next in flight of ideas, whereas the derailments in the speech of patients with Schizophrenia are much less understandable. Although this distinction may be helpful in the most classic cases, at the boundary there are many instances in which it is difficult or impossible to distinguish between loosening of associations and flight of ideas. Similarly, whereas rapid or pressured speech is often characteristic of mania, the speech of an excited or agitated patient with Schizophrenia may also be overwhelming. Therefore, it is best to base the differential diagnosis between Schizophrenic and Manic Episodes on the accompanying symptoms and overall course rather than on an isolated evaluation of the speech pattern.

The decision tree also includes the differential diagnosis for several disorders that are characterized by unusual speech first presenting itself in infancy, childhood, or adolescence. Symptoms such as difficulty understanding words, sentences, or specific types of words; having a markedly limited vocabulary; and having difficulty producing sentences may warrant a diagnosis of Expressive or Mixed Receptive-Expressive Language Disorder. In contrast, the speech in Autistic Disorder is characterized by stereotyped, repetitive, or idiosyncratic language usage. Inappropriate vocal outbursts that occur in the context of otherwise normal speech suggest a Tic Disorder.

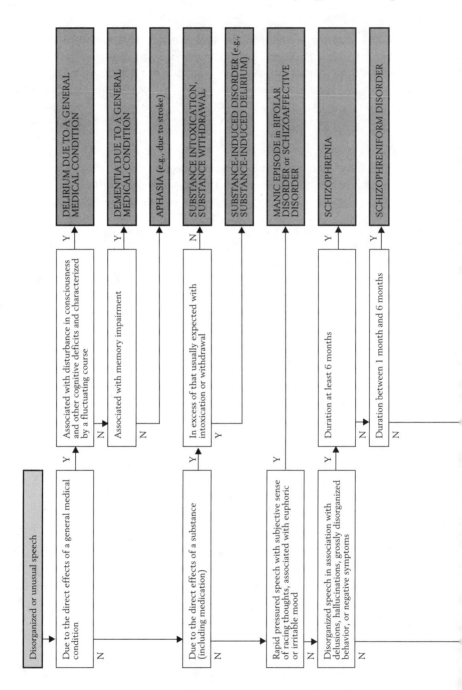

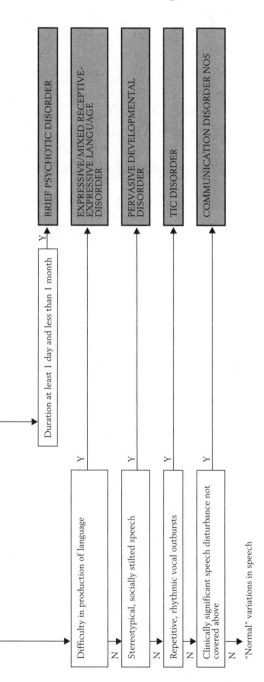

Decision Tree for Distractibility

Distractibility refers to an inability to filter out extraneous stimuli when attempting to concentrate on a particular task or activity. This is a very nonspecific symptom that occurs in a wide variety of mental disorders as well as in individuals without any mental disorder. The differential diagnosis rests on the age at onset, severity, the symptoms with which the distractibility is associated, and whether it results from a reaction to an external stressor. Clinically significant inattention with an onset in early childhood suggests a diagnosis of Attention-Deficit/Hyperactivity Disorder. Inattention with onset in adolescence suggests a variety of possible disorders, including recurrent Substance Intoxication or Withdrawal, Mood Disorder, and Schizophrenia. When inattention has a first onset later in life, it is especially important to consider the possible etiological role of a medication, drug of abuse, or a general medical condition.

You should consider a diagnosis of Delirium when inattention is severe and is associated with other cognitive or perceptual symptoms (e.g., disorientation, hallucinations). The hallmark of Delirium is a clouding of consciousness—the patient is unable to appreciate or respond appropriately to the external environment, to filter out irrelevant stimuli, and to follow instructions or reply to questions. Because Delirium is often a medical emergency, it is crucial to identify (and then correct) the underlying etiological factors that may be related to a general medical condition, substance use (including medication side effects), or some combination of these.

Distractibility is rarely the presenting symptom in disorders other than Attention-Deficit/Hyperactivity Disorder and Delirium. The evaluation of the differential diagnosis depends on what the accompanying features are (e.g., elevated mood in Manic Episode, excessive worry in Generalized Anxiety Disorder, persistent psychotic symptoms in Schizophrenia). It is also always useful to determine whether the patient has experienced psychosocial stressors that may be causing or increasing distractibility.

Finally, all of us (including the authors of this book) have differing abilities to filter out extraneous stimuli from the environment. Moreover, the nature and level of stimulation characteristic of the environment can increase or reduce any individual's ability to maintain attention. Whether a particular manifestation of distractibility constitutes an aspect of a mental disorder or should be considered within the normal range depends on its severity, persistence, and whether it causes clinically significant distress or impairment.

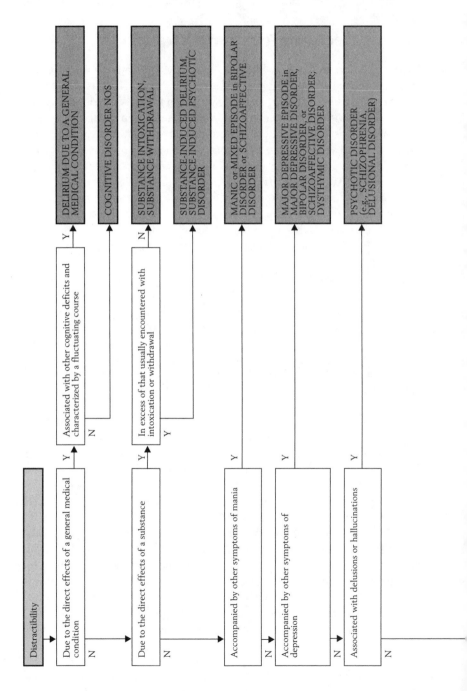

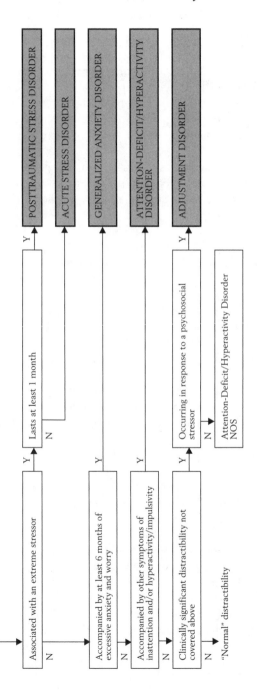

Decision Tree for Elevated or Irritable Mood

Most people (if they are at all lucky) have at least occasional moments when their mood is elevated and they feel at least slightly euphoric. And, sad to say, all of us can become more or less irritable under the right set of circumstances (e.g., not enough sleep, caught in traffic, under deadline pressure). This tree is not meant to apply to everyday experiences of elevated, expansive, or irritable mood.

The first step in the differential diagnosis is to ensure that the mood disturbance is not caused by a general medical condition or substance use. The first reflex, particularly for any late onset of these symptoms, should be to conduct a thorough medical workup and to evaluate whether the individual is using any medication (or drugs of abuse) that may produce mood changes as a side effect. In younger individuals, there is always a strong possibility that the changes in mood are caused by the effects of substance intoxication or withdrawal.

The next step is to determine whether the elevated or irritable mood is part of a Mood Episode (e.g., Manic, Hypomanic, or Mixed Episode). These episodes are not coded separately in DSM-IV-TR but instead form the building blocks for the Bipolar Disorders. It should be noted that the symptomatic definitions of Manic and Hypomanic Episode are essentially the same. The boundary between them depends on a clinical judgment as to the severity and impairment caused by the mood disturbance. By definition, a Hypomanic Episode does not cause marked impairment or distress and may even be compatible with improved social and job performance. In contrast to a Manic Episode, a Mixed Episode consists of a period of at least a week in which the criteria are simultaneously met for a Manic Episode and Major Depressive Episode.

The Bipolar Disorders are made up of combinations of Manic, Hypomanic, and Major Depressive Episodes. Bipolar I Disorder consists of one or more Manic Episodes and (optionally) one or more Major Depressive Episodes. The term *bipolar* is used even for individuals who have had just *unipolar* manic episodes (with no depressive episodes) because the vast majority of such individuals will eventually go on to have Major Depressive Episodes and their course, family loading, and treatment issues are equivalent to those who have had both Manic and Major Depressive Episodes. Bipolar II Disorder consists of one or more Major Depressive Episodes with intercurrent Hypomanic Episodes. Bipolar II Disorder, one of the few new diagnoses in DSM-IV, was introduced because of its treatment implications (i.e., the need to be cautious in the use of antidepressant medications in the absence of a mood stabilizer). Cyclothymic Disorder is a relatively uncommon bipolar spectrum disorder characterized by the alternation between periods of hypomania and depression that are less severe than a Manic or Major Depressive Episode.

Borderline Personality Disorder is included in this decision tree because individuals with this personality disorder certainly present with a persistent pattern of labile and irritable mood. However, if anything there is a tendency to overdiagnose Borderline Personality Disorder in patients who are in the midst of a mood episode. All too often, clinicians tend to label as "borderline" those Bipolar Disorder patients who are demanding, irritable, and irritating. The diagnosis of Borderline Personality Disorder requires that there have been an early onset and a persistent pattern that is not restricted to discrete mood episodes. Similarly, individuals in a Manic Episode who are disinhibited and have a low frustration tolerance may engage in antisocial acts that should not be confused with the long-term pattern of such behaviors in Antisocial Personality Disorder.

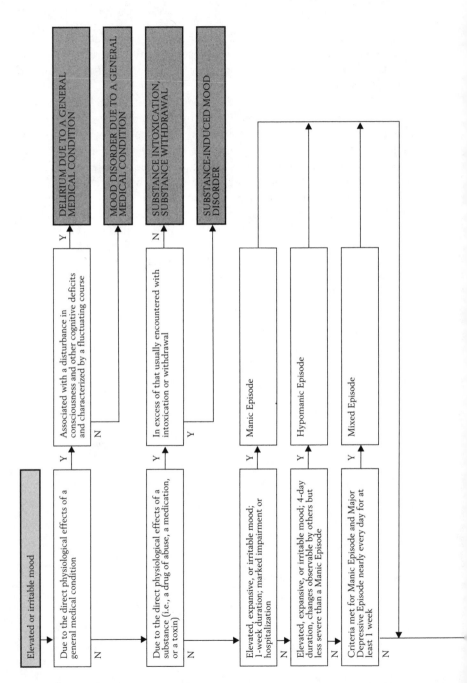

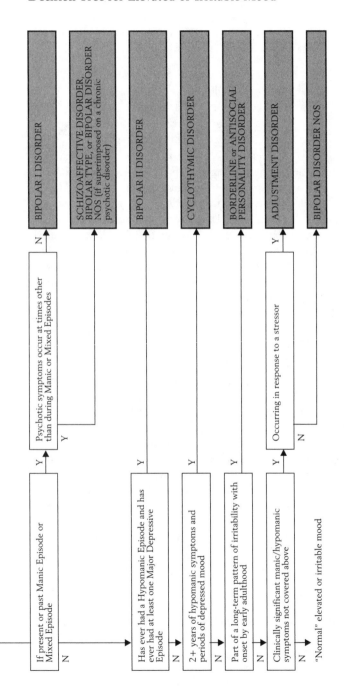

Decision Tree for Hallucinations

Hallucinations are sensory perceptions without external stimulation. When trying to determine the etiology of an hallucination, it is important to consider the sensory modality involved (i.e., whether the hallucinations are auditory, visual, gustatory, olfactory, or tactile). As a rule of thumb, visual, gustatory, and olfactory hallucinations are especially suggestive of an etiological general medical condition or substance and demand a careful medical workup. Similarly, a late age at first onset of hallucinations in any modality suggests the need for an especially careful medical workup. After ruling out a general medical condition or substance as an etiological factor, you must consider whether the hallucination is indicative of a psychotic disorder. There are four circumstances in which "hallucinations" should not count toward the diagnosis of a Psychotic Disorder: 1) those that occur in the context of Conversion Disorder or Somatization Disorder (so-called pseudohallucinations), which tend to affect multiple sensory modalities at the same time and to have psychologically meaningful content presented to the clinician in the form of an interesting story; 2) hallucinatory experiences that are part of a religious ritual or are a culturally sanctioned experience (e.g., hearing the voice of a dead relative giving advice); 3) those substance-induced hallucinations that occur with intact reality testing (e.g., an individual who is aware that the perceptual disturbances is due to recent hallucinogen use); and 4) hypnopompic or hypnagogic hallucinations that occur at the beginning or end of sleep episodes.

The content of hallucinations does not distinguish between a Mood Disorder With Psychotic Features and a nonmood psychotic disorder (e.g., Schizophrenia). This differential depends on the temporal relationship between the hallucinations and the mood disturbance. Hallucinations that occur exclusively during the mood episodes are considered part of a psychotic mood disorder, whereas hallucinations that occur when there are no mood symptoms or when the mood symptoms have remitted suggest Schizophrenia or Schizoaffective Disorder. Hallucinations that are features of a Mood Disorder With Psychotic Features can be mood-congruent (e.g., castigating accusatory voices in an individual with depression) or mood-incongruent (i.e., hallucinations that have nothing to do with the prevailing mood).

Illusions differ from hallucinations in that there is a misperception of an actual stimulus. When illusions occur in the absence of hallucinations, they do not count toward a diagnosis of a Psychotic Disorder and instead suggest Delirium, Substance Intoxication or Withdrawal, Schizotypal Personality Disorder, or no mental disorder.

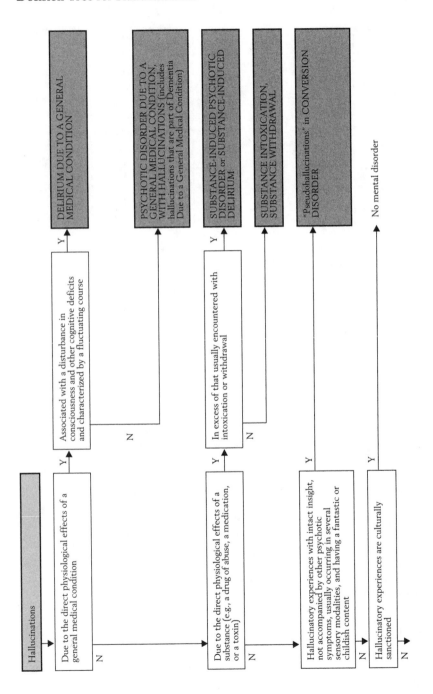

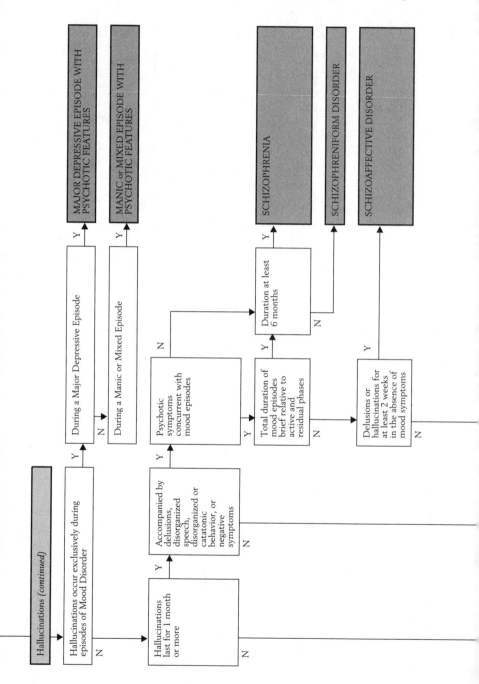

Decision Tree for Hypersomnia

Hypersomnia is defined as excessive sleepiness evidenced by prolonged sleep episodes or excessive daytime sleep that occurs almost daily. It should be noted that a diagnosis of Hypersomnia should be considered only if the person has been regularly getting adequate amounts of sleep—individuals would not qualify for this diagnosis if they are sleep deprived either because of insomnia or to accommodate their overscheduled lives. Drugs of abuse and many prescribed and over-the-counter medications have Hypersomnia as a significant side effect. For drugs of abuse, typically a diagnosis of Substance Intoxication or Withdrawal will suffice to cover the Hypersomnia. A diagnosis of Substance-Induced Sleep Disorder should be considered only if the Hypersomnia warrants independent clinical attention and is in excess of what one would expect given the substance used. A diagnosis of Substance-Induced Sleep Disorder can also be given for clinically notable Hypersomnia related to medications.

You must then rule out a general medical condition as the cause of the Hypersomnia. Breathing-Related Sleep Disorder (e.g., sleep apnea) is the most commonly diagnosed general medical condition responsible for sleep problems. However, because of their special differential diagnostic significance, DSM-IV-TR provides separate codes and descriptions for Breathing-Related Sleep Disorder and Narcolepsy rather than including them under Sleep Disorder Due to a General Medical Condition. Delirium should also be considered because it is so frequently associated with sleep disturbance.

The next step in the assessment is to consider whether the Hypersomnia is actually a symptom of another mental disorder. A number of mental disorders may include prominent symptoms of Hypersomnia, especially the "atypical" types of depressive episodes seen in Major Depressive Disorder and Bipolar I and II Disorders. A separate diagnosis of Hypersomnia Related to Another Mental Disorder should be considered only if the Hypersomnia is sufficiently severe to be a focus of independent clinical attention. Excessive daytime sleepiness may also be a feature of some specific sleep disorders, such as Parasomnias, and Circadian Rhythm Sleep Disorder. In such cases, a separate diagnosis of primary Hypersomnia is not given. The placement of primary Hypersomnia toward the end of this decision tree is meant to highlight its role as a diagnosis of exclusion that can be diagnosed only after all of the other more specific causes of Hypersomnia have been ruled out.

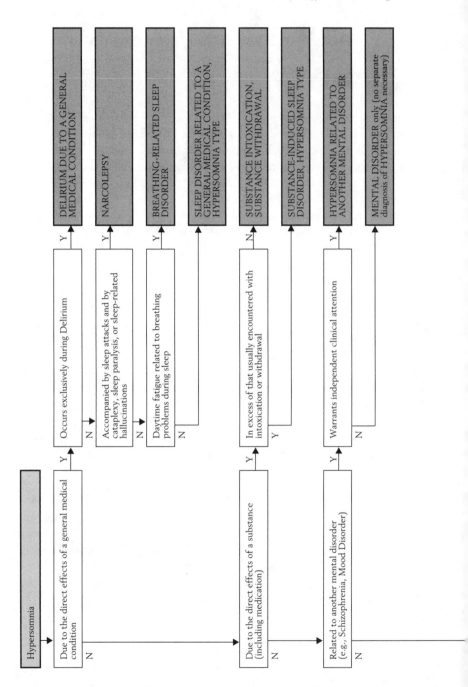

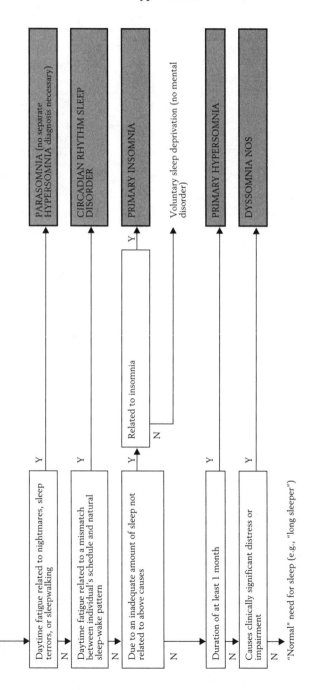

Decision Tree for Impulsivity

Impulsive behavior is a fairly nonspecific complication of a number of the psychiatric disorders that often requires the most urgent diagnostic and treatment attention because it may lead to considerable morbidity and mortality. However, it must be recognized that some degree of "impulsivity" is normal (and even desirable). Indeed, a total lack of spontaneity is itself considered a symptom of several disorders (e.g., Schizophrenia, Obsessive-Compulsive Personality Disorder). To be considered part of a mental disorder, the impulsivity must be persistent, severe, and lead to clinically significant impairment or distress. We also caution against the current tendency to "medicalize" impulsive behavior and to regard it as a manifestation of mental illness. Many quite extreme examples of loss of impulse control (e.g., murder) are not necessarily indicative of a mental disorder and may simply represent criminal behavior.

Substance use is perhaps the most common and devastating cause of impulsivity in our society and must be considered as a possible sole or contributory factor in every presentation of impulsive behavior. General medical conditions can also result in the disinhibition of impulse control, which is often accompanied by poor judgment and other cognitive symptoms warranting a diagnosis of Delirium or Dementia. When a general medical condition results in impulsivity that occurs in the absence of clinically significant cognitive impairment, the diagnosis is Personality Change Due to a General Medical Condition (usually of the Disinhibited or Aggressive Type).

Certain disorders are characterized by impulsivity that is confined exclusively to the episode of the disturbance. Once substance use and a general medical condition are ruled out, the next step is to determine whether the presentation includes symptoms that would lead to a diagnosis of a Mood Disorder, Schizophrenia, or one of the other psychotic disorders. Generalized impulsivity that has an early onset and persistent course is most likely to be associated with Attention-Deficit/Hyperactivity Disorder, Conduct Disorder, Antisocial Personality Disorder, or Borderline Personality Disorder. Other disorders are characterized by specific behaviors that can be conceptualized as an impairment in impulse control: Paraphilias, Eating Disorders, Substance Dependence, Pathological Gambling, and Intermittent Explosive Disorder.

DSM-IV-TR has a residual section for Impulse-Control Disorders Not Classified Elsewhere that includes Kleptomania, Pyromania, and Trichotillomania. The unifying construct for these disorders is an impaired ability to control the specific impulse (e.g., stealing, fire setting, or hair pulling) that follows a characteristic pattern. The individual experiences a sense of tension, followed by a feeling of pleasure or relief of tension once the act is committed. Thus, DSM-IV-TR distinguishes impulsive behavior in which the motive is pleasure or tension release from compulsive behavior (as in Obsessive-Compulsive Disorder) in which the motivation is reduction of distress or anxiety. In practice, however, it is often difficult to distinguish between tension release and anxiety reduction, and the boundary between the constructs of impulsive and compulsive behavior is far from clear. This ambiguity is reflected in the incorrect colloquial use of the word *compulsive* for behaviors that are usually considered to be *impulsive* such as *compulsive* gambling, eating, drug taking, spending, or sexual behavior.

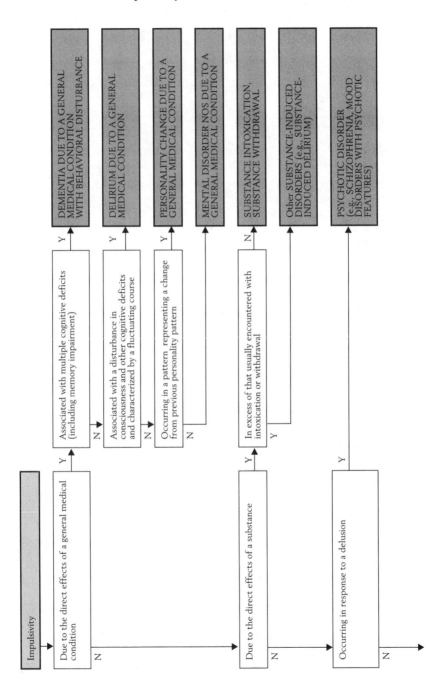

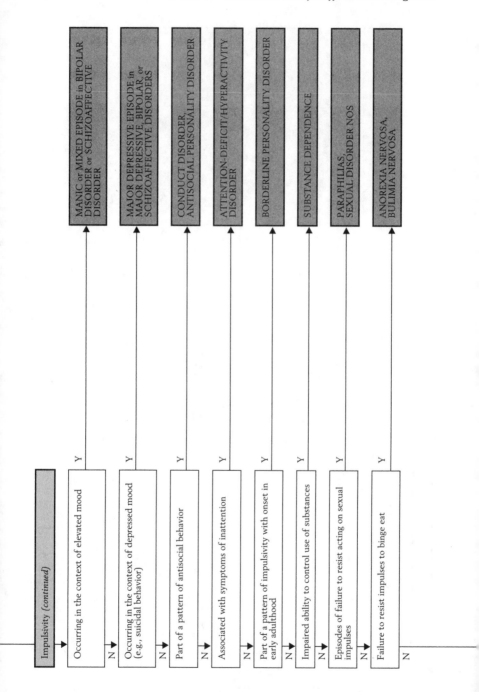

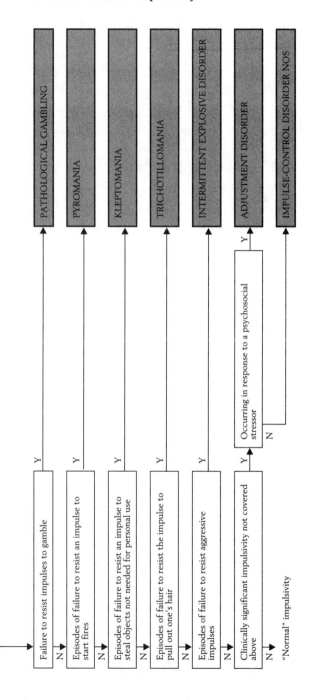

Decision Tree for Insomnia

Insomnia is defined in DSM-IV-TR as "difficulty falling or staying asleep or poor sleep quality." After ruling out a general medical condition or substance use (especially caffeine, alcohol, or medications) as the cause of the insomnia, you should consider whether the insomnia is actually a symptom of another mental disorder. A number of mental disorders may include insomnia as a presenting symptom, especially Major Depressive Disorder, Bipolar I and II Disorders, Schizophrenia, Posttraumatic Stress Disorder, and other Anxiety Disorders. A separate diagnosis of Insomnia Related to Another Mental Disorder in addition to the diagnosis of the more pervasive mental disorder is usually not necessary and should be considered only if the insomnia is sufficiently severe to be a focus of independent clinical attention. Insomnia also may be a feature of the more specific sleep disorders (e.g., Parasomnias and Circadian Rhythm Sleep Disorder) and in such cases is not given a separate diagnosis.

As with Primary Hypersomnia, the placement of Primary Insomnia toward the end of this decision tree highlights its role as a diagnosis of exclusion that can only be diagnosed after all other causes of insomnia have been ruled out. Frequently, individuals with Primary Insomnia have poor sleep hygiene (e.g., naps during the day, caffeine or stimulating activities before bedtime) and/or have developed a conditioned fear that they will not be able to sleep in their bed.

Some difficulty falling asleep (or maintaining sleep) is to be expected in everyone's life, especially in association with psychosocial stressors and as part of advancing age. Insomnia should only be considered as part of a mental disorder if the insomnia is severe, prolonged, and results in clinically significant distress or impairment.

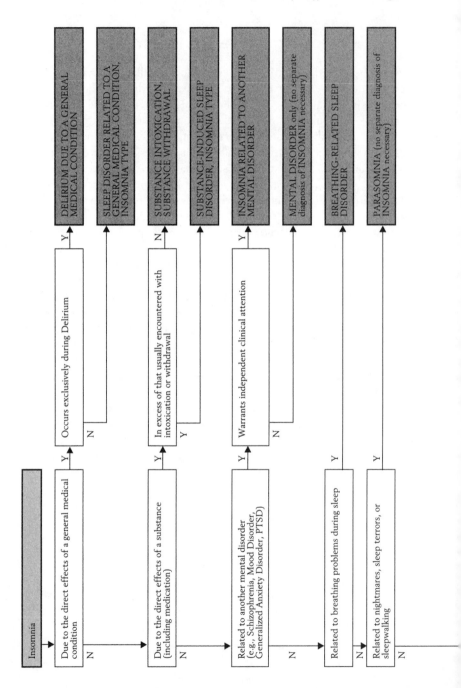

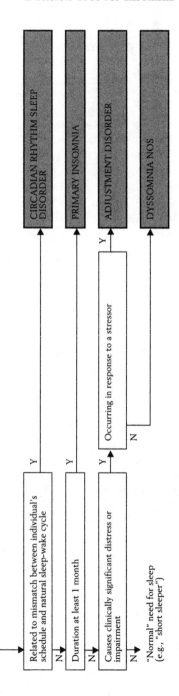

Decision Tree for Memory Impairment

Memory impairment can be characterized by difficulty in laying down new memories and/or in the recall of previous memories. The various aspects of memory functioning may be tested separately. These include 1) registration (the ability of the patient to repeat numbers or words immediately after hearing them), 2) short-term recall (the ability of the patient to repeat the names of three unrelated objects after a period of several minutes), 3) recognition (the ability of the patient to retrieve previously forgotten names if provided with clues), and 4) remote memory (the ability of the patient to recall important personal or historical events). The differential decisions in this tree concern whether the etiology of the memory loss is the direct physiological effect on the CNS of a general medical condition or substance use, whether it is an associated feature of another mental disorder, or whether the memory loss is a dissociative phenomenon (e.g., as in Posttraumatic Stress Disorder or one of the Dissociative Disorders).

Memory impairment is a defining feature of Delirium, Dementia, and Amnestic Disorder Due to General Medical Condition. These three disorders are differentiated based their accompanying symptoms. The hallmark of Delirium is a clouding of consciousness in which that patient is unable to appropriately maintain or shift attention. In Dementia, the memory impairment must be severe and accompanied by other clinically significant cognitive impairments (i.e., aphasia, apraxia, agnosia, or a disturbance in executive functioning). Memory impairment in the absence of other clinically significant cognitive deficits suggests a diagnosis of Amnestic Disorder. Memory impairment associated with substance use can either be temporary (as in Substance Intoxication, Substance Withdrawal, Substance-Induced Delirium, and Adverse Effects of Medication NOS) or permanent (as in Substance-Induced Persisting Dementia and Persisting Amnestic Disorder).

Memory impairment is also a common associated feature of a number of mental disorders. For example, memory impairment occurring in the context of a Major Depressive Episode can be so severe so as to resemble an irreversible dementing process. Frequently it is only when the memory impairment resolves after antidepressant treatment that it becomes clear that there was no comorbid Dementia. This differential is further complicated by the fact that the medication (e.g., lithium) being taken by the patient may also contribute to memory problems.

Dissociation is defined in the DSM-IV-TR glossary as a "disruption in the usually integrated functions of consciousness, memory, identity, or perception of the environment." Memory loss, especially for traumatic events, is a feature of each of the Dissociative Disorders as well as of Posttraumatic Stress Disorder and Acute Stress Disorder. Particularly when someone has been exposed to an event that is both physically and psychologically traumatic (e.g., car accident), it can be difficult to tease apart whether the memory loss is a psychological reaction to the events or is due to direct brain damage. Moreover, especially in forensic situations, feigned claims of memory loss may be used in an attempt to exonerate oneself from responsibility.

It should also be noted that virtually everyone wishes that his or her memory were better than it is and that this longing usually becomes more poignant as people get older and begin to find it more difficult to command their memories. Before considering the disorders on this decision tree, it must be determined that the memory loss is sufficiently severe so as to be clinically significant and that it is more severe than might be expected given the person's previous memory functioning and the norms for that person's age. In situations in which one wants to note reduced memory functioning that is nonetheless "normal" for the individual's age, Age-Associated Cognitive Decline (in the Other Conditions That May Be a Focus of Clinical Attention section) can be noted.

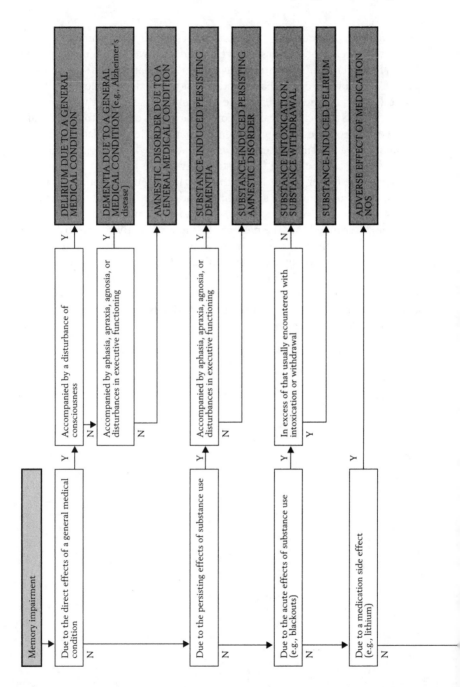

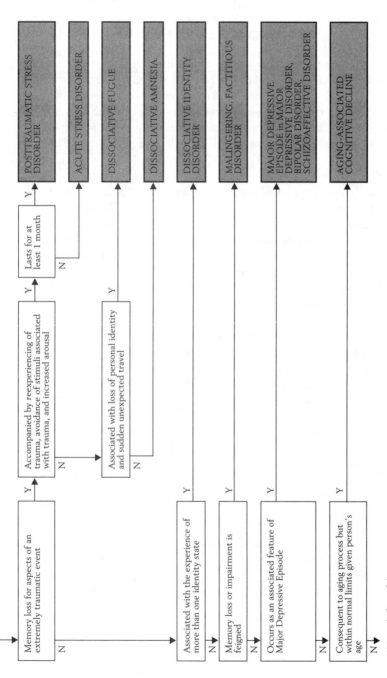

Decision Tree for Pain

Pain is a ubiquitous phenomenon in human life and disease but does not usually reach a sufficient level of severity or duration to warrant a separate diagnosis. The first step in the evaluation of pain is to determine whether a mental disorder diagnosis is appropriate to describe some aspect of the presentation. At any given moment, many patients in medical/surgical settings may be experiencing pain, and many will be receiving medication for it. The DSM-IV-TR diagnosis of Pain Disorder should be reserved only for those patients for whom psychological factors play an important role in the pathogenesis of the pain. Otherwise, the diagnosis of Pain Disorder Associated With a General Medical Condition (coded on Axis III) may apply. This is not considered to be a mental disorder and is listed alongside the other types of Pain Disorder in DSM-IV-TR only for completeness of differential diagnosis and because such individuals may benefit from treatments delivered by mental health professionals.

DSM-IV-TR includes two subtypes of Pain Disorder to allow the clinician to indicate the relative contribution of physical and psychological factors to the etiology of the Pain Disorder. Pain Disorder Associated With Psychological Factors describes those situations in which either there is no known medical condition accounting for the pain or any concurrent medical condition does not play a major role in its onset, severity, exacerbation, or maintenance. Pain Disorder Associated With Both Psychological Factors and a General Medical Condition is for those many cases encountered in mental health practice in which some combination of both physical and psychological factors are present and contribute to the etiology of the pain.

Because pain is a common associated feature of other DSM-IV-TR disorders (e.g., Major Depressive Disorder), Pain Disorder is not given as a separate diagnosis unless it is unusually severe, persistent, and becomes a main focus of clinical attention. Pain Disorder is not meant to be diagnosed if the pain symptoms are covered by the a diagnosis of Somatization Disorder or Dyspareunia.

Very often, individuals with Factitious Disorder or Malingering present with pain symptoms. The differential diagnosis between Pain Disorder and Factitious Disorder and Malingering may be especially difficult because it is often necessary to rely entirely on the patient's reporting of symptoms.

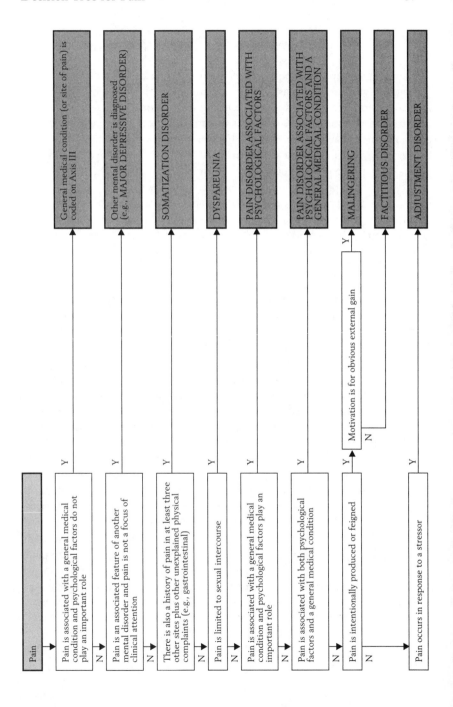

Decision Tree for Panic Attacks

Panic attacks are discrete episodes of intense fear or discomfort accompanied by symptoms such as palpitations, shortness of breath, sweating, trembling, derealization, and a fear of losing control or dying. Although panic attacks are required for a diagnosis of Panic Disorder, they also occur in association with a number of other DSM-IV-TR disorders listed in the tree. For example, if a patient with a snake phobia goes on a hike and steps on a snake, that experience could easily result in a panic attack that would be indicative of a Specific Phobia rather than Panic Disorder.

The first step in the differential for a panic attack is to rule out the presence of a general medical condition (e.g., hyperthyroidism or a pheochromocytoma) that would suggest the diagnosis of Anxiety Disorder Due to a General Medical Condition. Although mitral valve prolapse appears to be more frequent in individuals with panic attacks, a direct etiological connection has not yet been established. Therefore, an individual with mitral valve prolapse and panic attacks is considered to have a primary Panic Disorder. A number of substances, when taken in high enough doses or during withdrawal, can lead to a panic attack. Because caffeine is a common but covert culprit in this regard, taking a careful history of the consumption of caffeine-containing substances is important. If the panic attacks are a focus of separate clinical attention, Substance-Induced Anxiety Disorder should be diagnosed; otherwise, a diagnosis of Substance Intoxication or Withdrawal will suffice. Sometimes, individuals have their first panic attack while taking a substance and then go on to have additional attacks even when they are not taking any substance. Such subsequent attacks should not considered substance-induced but instead might warrant a diagnosis of Panic Disorder.

Once it is clear that the panic attacks are not the direct physiological consequence of a substance or general medical condition, the next step is to determine the relationship between the panic attacks and a possible situational trigger. By definition, at least two of the panic attacks in Panic Disorder are unexpected, that is, there is no relationship between the attacks and a situational cue (i.e., they arise "out of the blue"). In contrast, the panic attacks that occur in Social Phobia, Specific Phobia, Obsessive-Compulsive Disorder, and Posttraumatic Stress Disorder are closely related to the pertinent situational trigger (e.g., social situations such as public speaking, a specific situation such as closed places, obsessive concerns such as contamination fears, or reminders of the extreme stressor). If the panic attacks are not a component of a specific DSM-IV-TR disorder but nonetheless are judged to be clinically significant, a diagnosis of Adjustment Disorder may be appropriate. Finally, it should be noted that the experience of having a single isolated panic attack (or a very occasional panic attack) is not unusual and by itself does not warrant a diagnosis of a mental disorder.

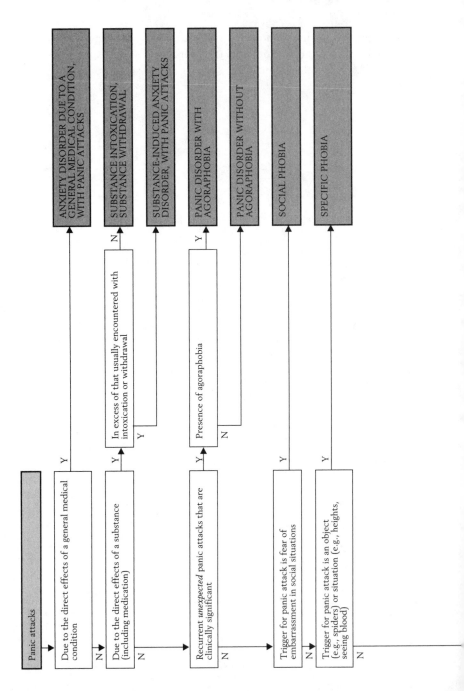

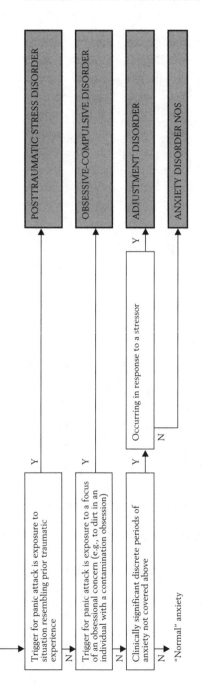

Decision Tree for Physical Complaints or Irrational Anxiety About Appearance

The problems covered in this decision tree are on the boundary between general medical conditions and mental disorders, and tend to receive insufficient attention from both fields. This may lead to misdiagnosis on both sides (sometimes with potentially tragic consequences); for example, an individual with Somatization Disorder may receive multiple unnecessary surgical procedures, whereas a patient with multiple sclerosis may be diagnosed as having Conversion Disorder. There are three ways of understanding unexplained physical symptoms: 1) that the symptoms are accounted for by an underlying general medical condition that has not yet manifested itself with clearly discernible objective findings (e.g., multiple sclerosis), 2) that the physical symptoms are best accounted for by a DSM-IV-TR disorder (e.g., Conversion Disorder, Panic Disorder, Major Depressive Disorder, Cocaine Withdrawal), or 3) that the physical symptoms are intentionally produced by the individual (i.e., Factitious Disorder, Malingering).

In determining whether an unexplained physical symptom is attributable to a Somatoform Disorder, the presence of a general medical condition must first be considered and ruled out. Contact with the patient's general medical provider is generally essential, as is a review of the patient's medical records. Ultimately, the determination of whether a general medical condition "fully" accounts for the patient's condition is an inherently imperfect judgment. Even if the clinician determines that the general medical condition accounts for the patient's symptoms, psychological factors could play a major role in the initiation and course of the illness and in the patient's response to treatment.

Clinicians often forget that individuals with a variety of other psychiatric disorders may, and very often do, present with a clinical picture that features their physical complaints. In fact, the appropriate DSM-IV-TR diagnosis is often missed either because the individual is so focussed on the physical symptoms or because the clinician overlooks the less obvious psychiatric symptoms that make up the full syndrome. Many cases of Major Depressive, Panic, Generalized Anxiety, and Substance Use Disorders presenting with physical symptoms are missed in this way, especially in primary care settings but also in mental health care settings. When an individual presents with atypical or unexplained physical symptoms, you must be particularly thorough in reviewing for the presence of pertinent DSM-IV-TR mental disorders. For example, for any individual presenting with unexplained shortness of breath, dizziness, and palpitations, it is crucial to ask whether the symptoms occur during discrete episodes of panic (see "Decision Tree for Panic").

The differential diagnosis with Factitious Disorder and Malingering rests on whether the patient is consciously feigning the symptoms. For example, an individual presents in the emergency room with a lower limb paralysis and stocking anesthesia that follows no known anatomical distribution. If this were Factitious Disorder or Malingering, the individual would be conscious of feigning the symptomatology (and, by the way, would probably feign a more convincing clinical picture based on reading medical textbooks). The diagnosis is more appropriately Conversion Disorder when the individual truly believes that the neurological symptoms are present and feels unable to move his leg. In practice, it can be difficult to evaluate these motivations and determine where they fall on the continuum between intentional feigning and unconscious symptom production.

The remainder of this decision tree depicts the relationship among the various Somatoform Disorders in DSM-IV-TR. Somatization Disorder is the most pervasive of the disorders (e.g., it requires a chronic pattern of complaints with at least four pain symptoms, two gastrointestinal symptoms, one sexual symptom, and one conversion symptom). Conversion Disorder, Pain Disorder, and Undifferentiated Somatoform Disorder cover more limited presentations and should not be diagnosed separately if criteria are also met for Somatization Disorder. Hypochondriasis is characterized more by preoccupation with the belief that there is an underlying serious illness rather than on the symptom itself. Body Dysmorphic Disorder is a pathological concern with the notion that one has a serious defect in physical appearance.

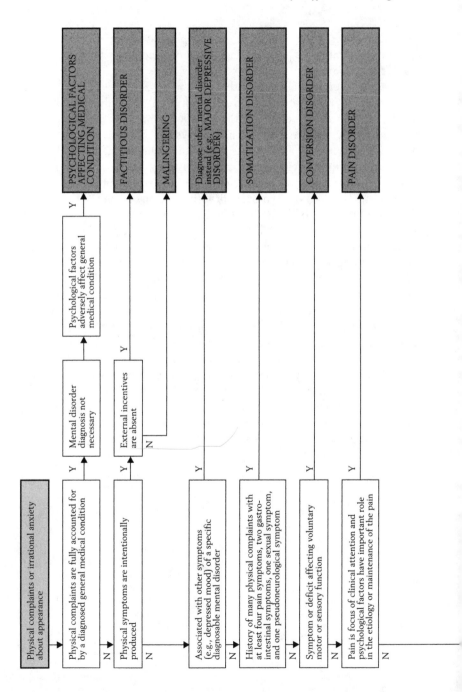

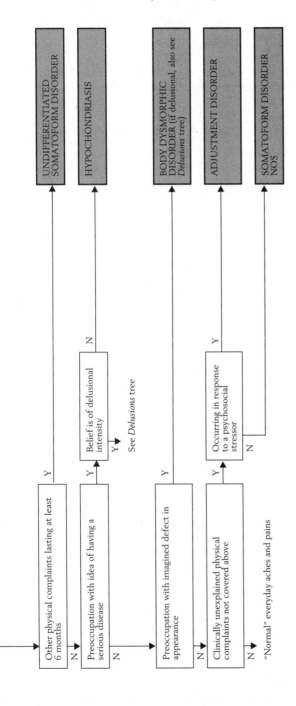

Decision Tree for Poor School Performance

Poor school performance is an all-too-common and very nonspecific aspect of childhood and adolescence. On the one hand, one should certainly not assume that every poor student has a mental disorder underlying his or her poor academic performance. On the other hand, most (if not all) mental disorders occurring in children may have a quite negative impact on school performance, and, not infrequently, difficulty in school is the chief complaint.

The evaluation for the causes of poor school performance will usually include testing for overall IQ and for deficits in specific academic skills (e.g., reading, mathematics, writing, expressive and receptive language). A definitive diagnosis of a DSM-IV-TR Developmental Disorder requires that the scores on an individually administered test be significantly below norms (e.g., two standard deviations). The next step is a careful assessment for the presence of the various psychiatric disorders that have impaired school performance as a consequence. This entails a careful history (supplemented by reports from parents, teachers, pediatricians), clinical observation, and an evaluation of the role of substance use. For example, are there clinically significant symptoms of inattention and/or hyperactive-impulsive behavior occurring in two or more different settings (as in Attention-Deficit/Hyperactivity Disorder)? Is there a pattern of antisocial behaviors such as truancy (as in Conduct Disorder)? Is there clinically significant depressed mood (as in Major Depressive Disorder)? Is there school refusal based on an inability to separate from attachment figures (as in Separation Anxiety Disorder)? and so forth. Because Developmental Disorders and other mental disorders frequently co-occur, it is important to evaluate for all possibilities in the tree and to make whichever diagnosis are appropriate.

The presence of a psychiatric disorder does not guarantee that it is the cause of school performance. Other factors (e.g., poor work habits, excessive TV watching, lack of motivation, poor schooling, disruptive home or community environment) may also play a significant role. Occasionally, the psychiatric disorder (e.g., Adjustment Disorder, Oppositional Defiant Disorder, Major Depressive Disorder) may be more the result of poor school performance than its cause.

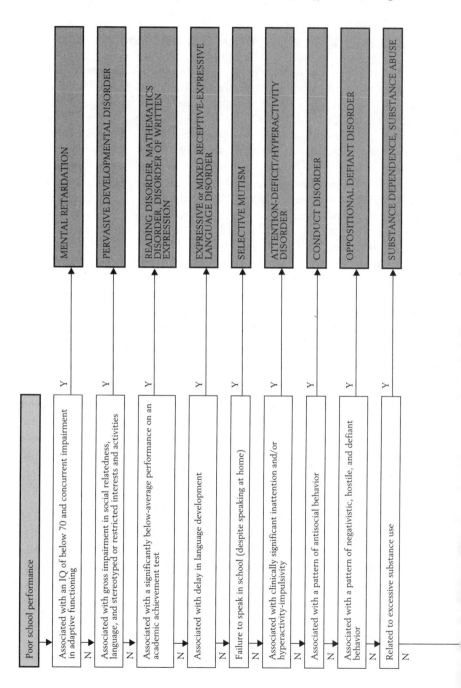

Poor school performance

Associated with an IQ of below 70 and concurrent impairment in adaptive functioning — Y → **MENTAL RETARDATION**

N

Associated with gross impairment in social relatedness, language, and stereotyped or restricted interests and activities — Y → **PERVASIVE DEVELOPMENTAL DISORDER**

N

Associated with a significantly below-average performance on an academic achievement test — Y → **READING DISORDER, MATHEMATICS DISORDER, DISORDER OF WRITTEN EXPRESSION**

N

Associated with delay in language development — Y → **EXPRESSIVE or MIXED RECEPTIVE-EXPRESSIVE LANGUAGE DISORDER**

N

Failure to speak in school (despite speaking at home) — Y → **SELECTIVE MUTISM**

N

Associated with clinically significant inattention and/or hyperactivity-impulsivity — Y → **ATTENTION-DEFICIT/HYPERACTIVITY DISORDER**

N

Associated with a pattern of antisocial behavior — Y → **CONDUCT DISORDER**

N

Associated with a pattern of negativistic, hostile, and defiant behavior — Y → **OPPOSITIONAL DEFIANT DISORDER**

N

Related to excessive substance use — Y → **SUBSTANCE DEPENDENCE, SUBSTANCE ABUSE**

N

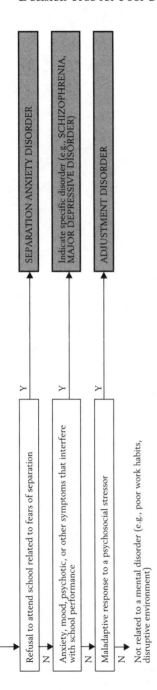

Refusal to attend school related to fears of separation — Y → SEPARATION ANXIETY DISORDER

N

Anxiety, mood, psychotic, or other symptoms that interfere with school performance — Y → Indicate specific disorder (e.g., SCHIZOPHRENIA, MAJOR DEPRESSIVE DISORDER)

N

Maladaptive response to a psychosocial stressor — Y → ADJUSTMENT DISORDER

N

Not related to a mental disorder (e.g., poor work habits, disruptive environment)

Decision Tree for Psychomotor Retardation

Psychomotor retardation is defined in the DSM-IV-TR Glossary as "visible generalized slowing of movements and speech." In its extreme form, psychomotor retardation may be characterized by unresponsiveness and mutism that is indistinguishable from catatonic stupor. The symptom of psychomotor retardation should be distinguished from other similar symptoms. Fatigue is a subjective sense of having decreased energy or being tired all the time but is not characterized by visible evidence of slowed movements. Leaden paralysis is the subjective sense that one's arms and legs are as "heavy as lead" and is a part of the "atypical" pattern of symptoms in a Major Depressive Episode. Avolition (one of the negative symptoms of Schizophrenia) is characterized by a lack of motivation to carry out behaviors rather than being physically slowed down.

General medical conditions may cause psychomotor retardation that usually does not warrant a separate mental disorder diagnosis. It is important to remember that psychomotor changes associated with Delirium go in both directions. Very few clinicians miss the dramatic presentations of Delirium associated with psychomotor agitation (e.g., the patient pulling out an intravenous line). The "quiet" cases of delirium associated with psychomotor retardation are much more likely to be unrecognized.

Another common "missed" cause of slowed movements is Neuroleptic-Induced Parkinsonism. This differentiation is complicated by the fact that a number of disorders for which neuroleptics are given can themselves present with psychomotor retardation (e.g., Schizophrenia, Mood Disorder With Psychotic Features, Delirium). A change in medication (e.g., reducing the neuroleptic dose or administering anticholinergic medication) often can be helpful in making the distinction.

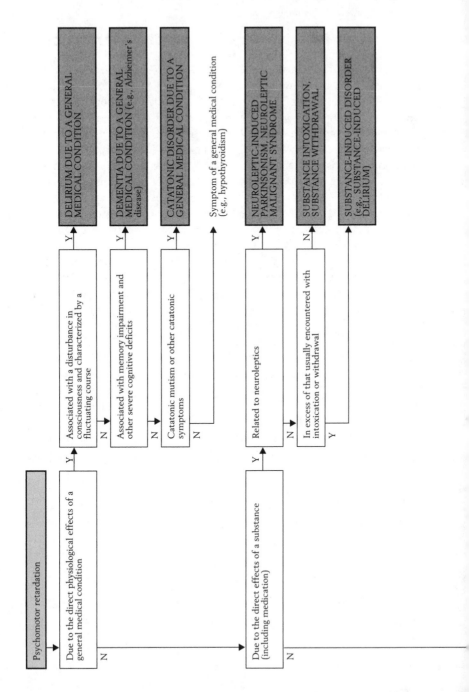

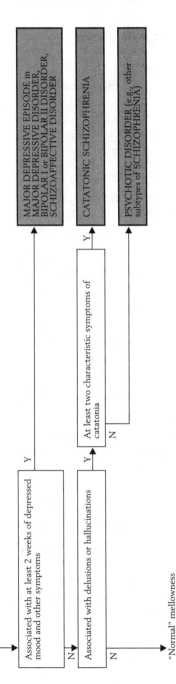

Decision Tree for Self-Mutilation

The types of self-mutilating behavior described in this tree include cutting, burning, head-banging, hair-pulling, skin-picking, self-biting, and hitting various parts of one's own body. It is of interest that the frequency of self-mutilation appears to be greatest in situations in which the individual is confined (e.g., hospitals, prisons, children's homes). This makes for interesting dilemmas when a patient who is about to be discharged from the hospital increases self-mutilating behaviors (that may in fact be reinforced by remaining in that setting).

The motivation for self-mutilation varies in the various diagnoses for which it is a complication. The most frequent diagnosis associated with self-mutilation is Borderline Personality Disorder. For some patients with this disorder, the self-mutilating behavior occurs as a means of "treating" dissociative states, and the patient returns to feeling alive only when experiencing pain or seeing blood. In others, self-mutilation is a means of "treating" intense dysphoria or counteracting intense anger. The likelihood of self-mutilative episodes is greatly increased by Substance Intoxication or Withdrawal. The motivation for self-mutilation in psychotic patients is usually a delusional belief (e.g., the need to punish evil spirits) or a response to a command hallucination. In Delirium and Dementia, the self-mutilation sometimes occurs as a by-product of the confusion (e.g., struggling against restraints). The self-mutilation that infrequently occurs as a complication of Obsessive-Compulsive Disorder results from the inability to resist the constant need to perform a compulsive act (e.g., cleaning hands raw as a result of hand-washing compulsion). In Trichotillomania, there is an inability to resist the impulse to pull out one's hair, which may result in patches of hair loss. In Sexual Masochism, the motivation for the self-mutilation is sexual pleasure.

Stereotypies, which may or may not result in self-injury, are a component of Stereotyped Movement Disorder, Mental Retardation, and Pervasive Developmental Disorders. When Stereotyped Movement Disorder results in clinically significant self-injury, this can be indicated by specifying With Self-Injurious Behavior. Stereotypies are not infrequent in Mental Retardation and should be diagnosed separately only if they are severe enough to be a focus of treatment. Because stereotypies are part of the criteria set for Pervasive Developmental Disorders, an additional diagnosis of Stereotypic Movement Disorder is not made.

Self-mutilating behavior is sometimes a manifestation of Factitious Disorder or Malingering. The patient learns that cutting or burning will result in a desired hospitalization or prevent an undesired discharge. Factitious Disorder and Malingering are differentiated based on the underlying motivation. In Malingering, the motivation is some obvious gain (e.g., getting medication), whereas the motivation in Factitious Disorder is the need to be taken care of.

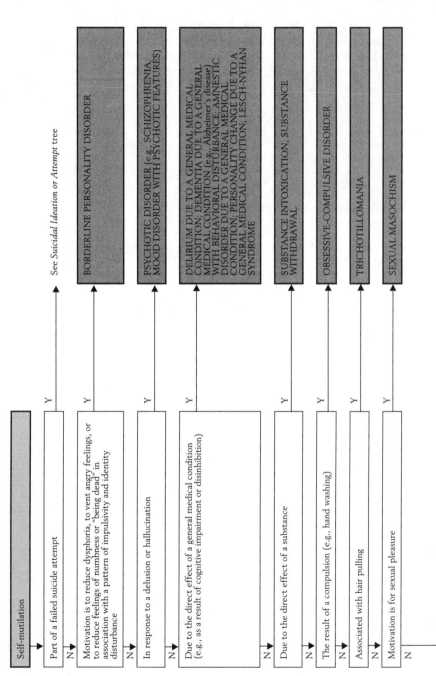

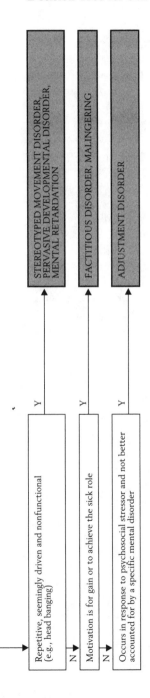

Repetitive, seemingly driven and nonfunctional (e.g., head banging)

Y → STEREOTYPED MOVEMENT DISORDER, PERVASIVE DEVELOPMENTAL DISORDER, MENTAL RETARDATION

N

Motivation is for gain or to achieve the sick role

Y → FACTITIOUS DISORDER, MALINGERING

N

Occurs in response to psychosocial stressor and not better accounted for by a specific mental disorder

Y → ADJUSTMENT DISORDER

Decision Tree for Sexual Dysfunction

The major difficulty in evaluating sexual dysfunctions is that there are no accepted guidelines for determining what is "normal" sexual functioning. The threshold for normal sexual functioning varies with the person's age, prior sexual experience, the availability and novelty of partners, and the expectations and standards characteristic of the person's cultural, ethnic, or religious group. Successful arousal and orgasm require a level of sexual stimulation that is adequate in focus, intensity, and duration. A diagnosis of an arousal disorder or orgasmic disorder therefore requires a clinical judgment that the person has experienced adequate stimulation. Moreover, it must be remembered that occasional sexual dysfunction is an inherent part of human sexuality and is not indicative of a disorder unless it is persistent or recurrent and results in marked distress or interpersonal difficulty.

Once the clinical judgment has been made that the sexual dysfunction is clinically significant, the next task is to determine its underlying etiology. The possible etiologies include psychological factors, general medical conditions, the side effects of many prescribed medications, and the consequence of drug abuse. This evaluation can be difficult because very often more than one etiology contributes to the sexual dysfunction. For example, it is not uncommon for someone who develops mild erectile dysfunction as a result of a general medical condition (e.g., vascular problems) to develop other sexual dysfunctions (e.g., low desire) as a psychological consequence. Before deciding that any sexual dysfunction is mediated strictly by psychological factors, it is important to consider the possible contribution of a medical condition or substance (including medication side effects), especially since these etiologies often have specific treatment implications (e.g., discontinuation of the offending medication). On the other hand, it is also important to remember that the identification of a specific etiologic general medical condition, medication, or drug of abuse does not negate the important contribution of psychological factors to the etiology of the dysfunction.

Sexual problems are also commonly associated with a number of mental disorders (e.g., Mood Disorders, Anxiety Disorders, Somatoform Disorders, Psychotic Disorders). An additional diagnosis of a Sexual Dysfunction is not given if the sexual problems are best attributed to an Axis I Disorder. For example, low sexual desire occurring only during a Major Depressive Episode should not receive a separate diagnosis of Hypoactive Sexual Desire Disorder. Both diagnoses can be given only if the low sexual desire is judged to be independent of the depressive disorder (i.e., it precedes the onset of the depressive episode or persists long after the depression has remitted).

The primary sexual dysfunctions are organized based on where during the sexual response cycle the problem occurs. Hypoactive Sexual Desire Disorder and Sexual Aversion Disorder are for problems related to the initial phase, Sexual Desire. Female Arousal Disorder and Male Erectile Disorder are for problems related to the second phase, Sexual Excitement. Female and Male Orgasmic Disorder and Premature Ejaculation are for problems related to the third phase, Orgasm. Not infrequently, problems occur in more than one phase of the sexual response cycle. Because the phases of the sexual response cycle occur in sequence, successful functioning in one phase generally requires successful functioning in the previous phases (e.g., orgasm requires some level of arousal, which requires some level of desire). However, anticipation of the recurrence of problems in a later phase (e.g., a man having difficulty ejaculating) often leads to problems in an earlier phase (e.g., consequent erectile dysfunction or low sexual desire). Finally, the tree concludes with two disorders covering physical discomfort that is related to sexual intercourse: Dyspareunia (pain occurring during intercourse) and Vaginismus (vaginal spasms that interfere with sexual intercourse).

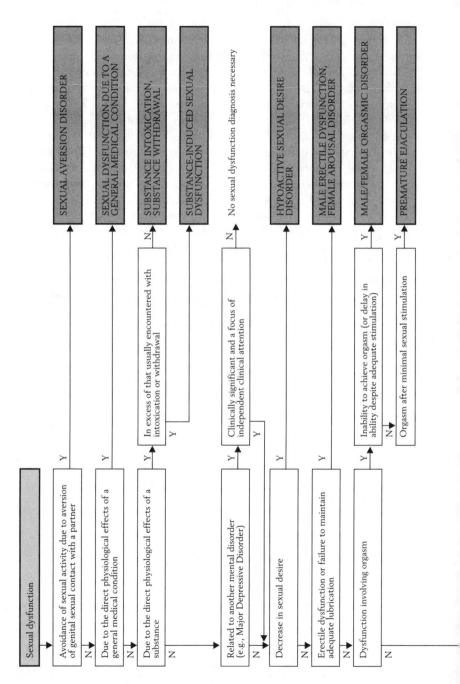

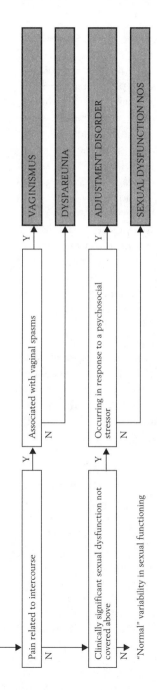

Decision Tree for Suicidal Ideation or Attempt

When evaluating suicidality, it is important to determine the urgency of current suicidal thoughts, the degree to which definite plans have been formulated and acted on, the availability of a means of suicide, the lethality of the method, the urgency of the impulse, the presence of psychotic symptoms, the history of previous suicidal thoughts and attempts, family history of suicidal behavior, and current and past substance use. The degree of suicidality is on a continuum ranging from recurrent wishes to be dead, to feelings that others would be better off if one were dead ("passive suicidal thoughts"), to formulating suicidal plans to overt suicidal behaviors.

Perhaps because suicidal behavior is a defining feature of a Major Depressive Episode, most people associate suicide most closely with Mood Disorders. Although certainly suicide is an important complication of mood disorders, as this tree illustrates, it must be considered in the management of a wide array of DSM-IV-TR disorders. Moreover, the risk of suicide increases dramatically when the individual has more than one disorder because each of these may independently contribute to the risk (e.g., a particularly common and dangerous combination includes Major Depressive Disorder, Alcohol Dependence, Borderline Personality Disorder).

Suicidal behavior may result from symptoms other than depressed mood. For example, suicidal behavior may occur under the direction of delusions or command hallucinations (as in Schizophrenia or Mood Disorder With Psychotic Features), may be related to confusion or other cognitive impairment (as in Delirium, Dementia, Substance Intoxication or Withdrawal), or may result from disinhibition (as in a Manic Episode, Substance Intoxication, or Antisocial Personality Disorder).

Borderline Personality Disorder and Antisocial Personality Disorder have a 5%-10% risk of successful suicide, perhaps resulting from the impulsivity, labile moods, low frustration tolerance, and high rates of substance use characteristic of such individuals. Similarly, Conduct Disorder is an important predictor of suicide in adolescents, particularly when it is accompanied by substance use and mood symptoms.

Some patients may consider suicide as a solution to what to them appears to be an intractable symptom (e.g., pain, insomnia, panic) or life problem (e.g., unemployment, divorce). The two clinical reflexes that should be triggered are the institution of aggressive treatment for the specific problem and an extensive evaluation for other complicating conditions (e.g., Major Depressive Disorder, Substance Abuse).

The evaluation of suicidal ideation or behavior must take into account the fact that such symptoms are often feigned as a way of gaining admission to the hospital or to solve other life problems. Patients quickly learn the power of saying the phrase, "I want to kill myself" as a way of influencing clinicians, family members, and other individuals important in their lives. In Malingering, the motivation is some obvious gain (e.g., getting transferred from prison to hospital, getting a place to spend the night). In contrast, the motivation in Factitious Disorder is a psychological need to assume the sick role, especially in individuals who are attempting to make the hospital their more or less permanent home.

Adjustment Disorder applies to those individuals who develop suicidal ideation or behavior in response to psychosocial stressors and in the absence of other symptoms that would be the criteria for a specific DSM-IV-TR disorder. This diagnosis is most commonly used to describe suicidal behavior in adolescents.

Although this is a controversial topic, it does seems to us that there are certain extreme circumstances (e.g., an intractable terminal illness) in which the desire to kill oneself does not necessarily represent a mental disorder. However, before arriving at this conclusion, it is crucial that there be a thorough evaluation to rule out all other more treatable causes of suicidal ideation (e.g., depression, pain, insomnia, psychosis, delirium).

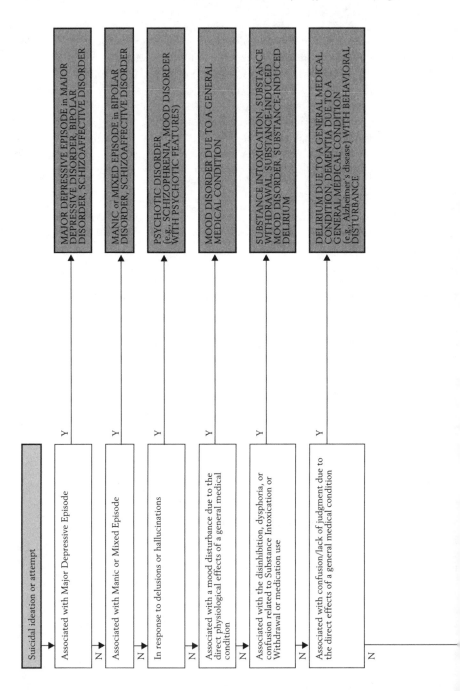

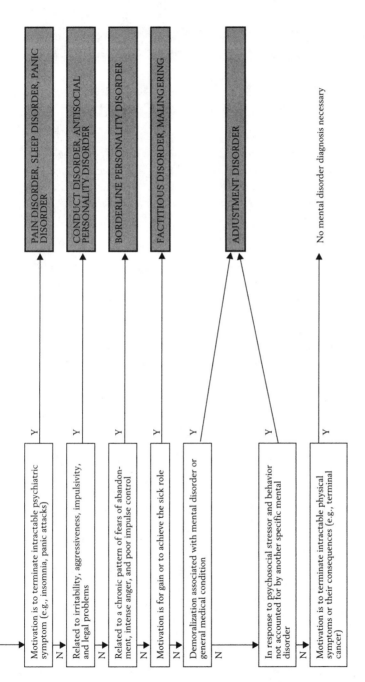

Trees Based on Presumed Etiology

Decision Tree for Mental Disorders Due to a General Medical Condition

It is a crucial part of the evaluation of every patient to consider the possibility that the symptoms are due to the direct physiological effect of a general medical condition (see "Step 3" in Chapter 1). In fact, psychiatric symptoms are sometimes the first harbingers of a not-yet-diagnosed general medical condition. Determining that a general medical condition is responsible for the psychopathology has obvious treatment implications—treatment of the general medical condition is itself important and often results in the remission of the psychiatric symptoms.

Not every behavioral symptom arising from a general medical condition warrants a diagnosis of a Mental Disorder Due to a General Medical Condition. Certainly, most patients who are a bit anxious, sad, fatigued, or having sleepless nights because of a general medical condition do not have a mental disorder that would be covered in this tree. The disorders in this tree should be considered only when the symptoms are sufficiently severe and prolonged to become an independent focus of clinical attention. Not uncommonly, the psychiatric presentation Due to a General Medical Condition is characterized by a mixture of symptoms from more than one section of the classification (e.g., mood, anxiety, and sleep). In most cases, you should choose the diagnosis that reflects the most prominent aspect of the symptom presentation.

Delirium Due to Multiple Etiologies and Dementia Due to Multiple Etiologies have been included in DSM-IV-TR (and in this tree) to emphasize that very often these conditions have multiple interacting etiologies. Moreover, the medications used to treat general medical conditions often have behavioral side effects that may be confused both with primary psychiatric symptoms and with the psychiatric manifestations of the general medical condition itself. This is particularly common in elderly individuals who may be taking a number of different medications and have a reduced ability to metabolize (or eliminate) them.

Finally, when communicating or recording the diagnosis, the actual name of the etiological general medical condition should be used on Axis I (e.g., 293.84 Mood Disorder Due to Hyperthyroidism, With Manic Features). Furthermore, the general medical condition should also be coded on

Axis III (e.g., 244.9 Hypothyroidism). To help ease your coding burden, DSM-IV-TR includes an appendix (Appendix G) of selected general medical codes.

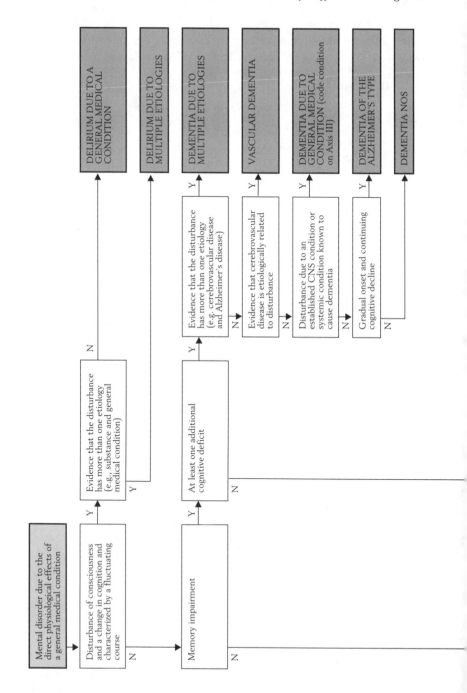

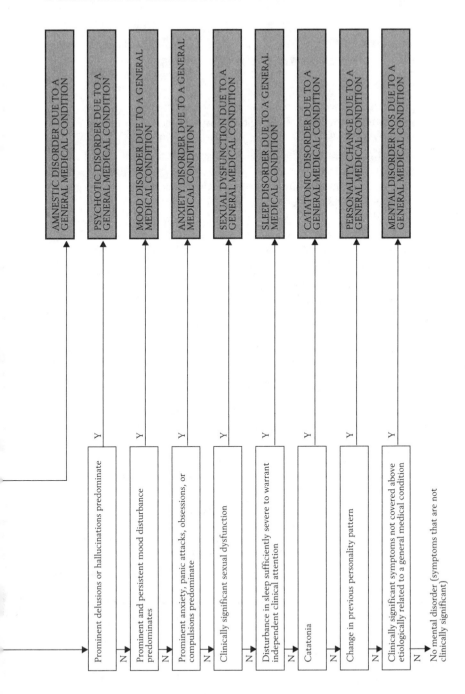

Decision Tree for Mental Disorder Due to Substance Use

Many individuals can take substances without having any clinically significant problems that would warrant a DSM-IV-TR diagnosis. However, Substance-Related Disorders are among the most common and impairing of the mental disorders. Because substance-related presentations are so frequently encountered in mental health, substance treatment, and primary care settings, a Substance-Related Disorder must be considered in every differential diagnosis. In our experience, these disorders are among the most frequently missed in clinical practice.

In DSM-IV-TR, the term *substance-related* refers to disorders associated with drugs of abuse, the side effects of medication, and toxin-induced states. There are two types of substance-related diagnoses in DSM-IV-TR: the Substance Use Disorders, which describe a pattern of problematic substance use (i.e., Substance Dependence and Substance Abuse); and the Substance-Induced Disorders, which describe behavioral syndromes that are caused by a direct effect of the substance on the CNS. This decision tree is confined to the Substance-Induced Disorders that are listed in the right-hand column of the tree. It should be noted that more often than not, Substance-Induced Disorders occur in the context of an accompanying Substance Use Disorder. When this occurs, both should be diagnosed (e.g., Alcohol Withdrawal and Alcohol Dependence).

Substance Intoxication and Substance Withdrawal can be characterized by psychopathology that mimics the other disorders contained in the rest of DSM-IV-TR and must always be considered in the differential diagnosis of every condition (see "Step 2" in Chapter 1). The other Substance-Induced Disorders (e.g., Substance-Induced Mood Disorder, Substance-Induced Persisting Dementia) have been included in DSM-IV-TR to diagnose substance-induced symptom presentations that are in excess of those usually encountered with the typical intoxication or withdrawal syndrome for that substance. Moreover, these specific substance-induced disorders should be diagnosed instead of Substance Intoxication or Withdrawal only if the symptoms warrant independent clinical attention. For example, virtually every individual withdrawing from cocaine will experience some dysphoric mood, and in most situations a diagnosis of Cocaine Withdrawal will suffice. However, were the individual to become suicidally depressed, the diagnosis of Cocaine-Induced Mood Disorder may be appropriate. Often more than one symptom (e.g., depressed mood and anxiety) may be prominent enough to be a focus of clinical attention. In such situations, it is generally preferable to give just the one substance-induced diagnosis indicating the predominating symptom.

The psychiatric sequelae to substance use can occur in any of four contexts: 1) as an acute effect of Substance Intoxication, 2) as an acute effect of Substance Withdrawal, 3) as a medication side effect not necessarily related to intoxication or withdrawal, and 4) as an effect that endures even after the substance is no longer present (a Substance-Induced Persisting Disorder). The term *persisting* indicates that the psychopathology results not from the acute effects of the substance or toxin but rather from the structural damage it has caused to the CNS. DSM-IV-TR includes three such disorders: Substance-Induced Persisting Dementia, Substance-Induced Persisting Amnestic Disorder, and Hallucinogen Persisting Perceptual Disorder.

Delirium Due to Multiple Etiologies and Dementia Due to Multiple Etiologies have been included in DSM-IV-TR (and in this tree) to emphasize that very often these conditions have multiple interacting etiologies. A common (and sometimes devastating error) is to assume your job is finished once you have identified a substance as a contributing etiology to the Delirium or Dementia and therefore to miss the associated contribution of the head trauma or other general medical conditions.

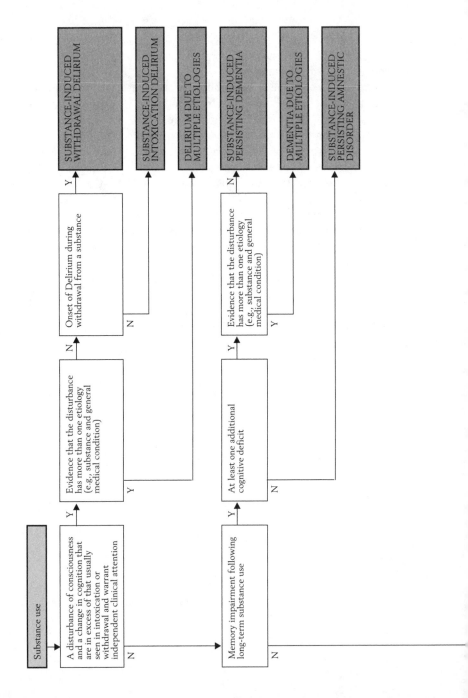

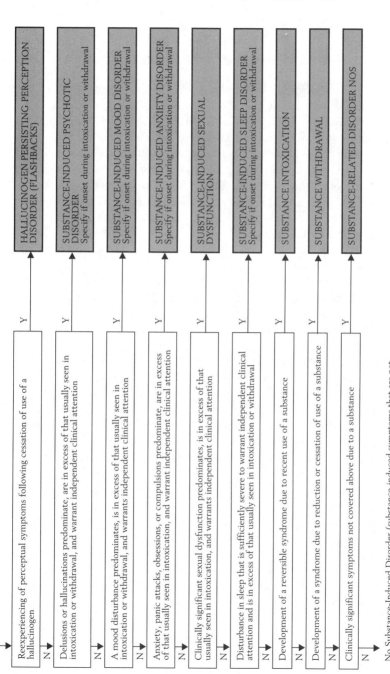

Decision Tree for
Mental Disorder Due to Stress

Psychosocial stressors are important in the pathogenesis of all of the DSM-IV-TR disorders, but their specific etiological role serves as a defining feature for only a few. There are two disorders in DSM-IV-TR that can be diagnosed only when the individual has been exposed to an extreme stressor. Posttraumatic Stress Disorder is characterized by a persistent reexperiencing of the stressful situation, the avoidance of stimuli recalling the event, and a pattern of increased arousal. Acute Stress Disorder is for similar reactions that last for less than 1 month occurring in the immediate aftermath of exposure to a stressor. If the reaction to an extreme stressor is of psychotic proportions, then the diagnosis of Brief Psychotic Disorder With Marked Stressors is made instead. Dissociative Amnesia is another disorder that may occur in response to a stressful experience.

Many clinicians are confused about the relationship between the Adjustment Disorders and the other conditions in DSM-IV-TR that are so often precipitated by the presence of a psychosocial stressor. Adjustment Disorder is diagnosed for those presentations in which the maladaptive response to the stressor causes clinically significant distress or impairment but does not meet the threshold requirements for any specific DSM-IV-TR disorder. In contrast, when the criteria are met for a specific DSM-IV-TR disorder, that disorder is diagnosed regardless of the presence or absence of associated stressors. For example, if a depressive reaction occurs in response to a job loss or learning that one has a serious illness, the diagnosis is Major Depressive Disorder if the reaction meets the full criteria for a Major Depressive Episode. A less severe, but nonetheless clinically significant, depressive reaction might instead be diagnosed as Adjustment Disorder With Depressed Mood. Axis IV is provided in DSM-IV-TR to allow specification of the stressor.

Bereavement is a reaction to a specific psychosocial stressor (i.e., loss of a loved one), but it is not considered to be a mental disorder because such reactions are considered to be "normal," even if clinically significant. When grieving is more severe or prolonged than is characteristic of Bereavement, then a diagnosis of Major Depressive Disorder (or Adjustment Disorder) may be more appropriate.

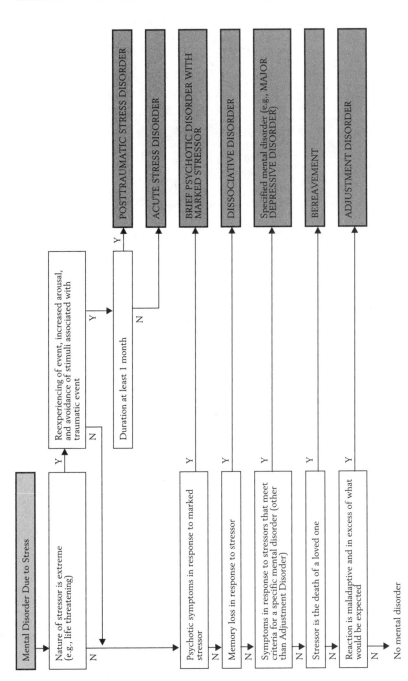

3

Differential Diagnosis
by the Tables

Differential diagnosis is at the heart of every initial clinical encounter and is the beginning of every treatment plan. The clinician must determine which conditions are possible candidates for consideration and then choose from among them the disorder that bests accounts for the presenting symptoms. The biggest problem encountered in differential diagnosis is the tendency for premature closure in coming to a final diagnosis. A number of studies have indicated that clinicians usually decide on the final diagnosis within the first 5 minutes of meeting the patient. Forming initial impressions can be valuable in helping to suggest which questions need to be asked and which hypotheses need to be tested. Unfortunately, however, often enough first impressions are wrong—particularly because the patient's current state may not be an accurate reflection of the longitudinal course. Accurate diagnosis requires a methodical consideration of all of the possible contenders in the differential diagnosis. The use of the differential diagnosis tables in this chapter will ensure that your evaluations are systematic and comprehensive.

Sixty-two tables have been provided covering the most important disorders in DSM-IV-TR. The "Table of Contents" provides a list of the differential diagnosis tables that have been included. Each table comprises two columns. The left-hand column lists the disorders that must be ruled out as part of the differential diagnosis of the disorder in question. The right-hand column suggests those distinguishing features that may be helpful in ruling out these contenders. Unless otherwise stated, if the criteria are fully met for both disorders, both should be diagnosed. We find that the best way to use the tables is to look over the disorders in the left-hand column to gain a "bird's-eye" view of the differential diagnostic task. The next step is a consideration of the specific features that characterize each of the individual disorders in the differential diagnosis.

We would also like to offer a few cautions about the use of the tables. You will note that the pertinent Not Otherwise Specified categories are not included in the differential diagnosis tables although they are an important consideration in the differential diagnosis for every disorder. Every experienced clinician knows that the complexity of practice offers many presentations that fall between the neatly defined DSM-IV-TR disorders. Many patients do not present a clear picture that comfortably approximates the prototype for any of the disorders described in the DSM-IV-TR criteria sets. Instead, patients often have clinical features that appear to be at the boundary between criteria sets or satisfy the criteria for a number of possibly related disorders. It is important to recognize that a boundary patient is a boundary patient and should not be shoehorned into a diagnosis that does not fit well. Such patients may require serial trials of treatment to help clarify the most appropriate diagnosis and plan of management.

Moreover, the differential diagnostic tables tend to focus on cross-sectional symptom presentations because these are the easiest to define and evaluate. Other factors that may be useful in guiding differential diagnosis include the patient's previous history, family history of psychopathology, course, biological test results, and responses to previous treatment trials. Especially in doubtful cases, these factors may tip the differential diagnostic balance one way or the other.

Disorders First Diagnosed in Infancy, Childhood, or Adolescence

Differential Diagnosis for Mental Retardation

Mental Retardation must be differentiated from . . .	In contrast to Mental Retardation, the other condition . . .
Learning Disorders	• Is characterized by an impairment confined to a specific area of academic achievement (i.e., reading, arithmetic, writing skills) rather than a general impairment in intellectual functioning.
Communication Disorders	• Is confined to speech or language impairment.
Pervasive Developmental Disorders	• Includes qualitative impairments in social skills and a restricted repertoire of interests or activities, although Mental Retardation is frequently comorbid.
Dementia	• Is characterized by a significant decline in intellectual functioning. Both Dementia and Mental Retardation can be diagnosed if onset is before age 18 years.
Borderline Intellectual Functioning	• Is characterized by a lesser degree of intellectual impairment (IQ above 70) or no problems in adaptive functioning if IQ is below 70.

Differential Diagnosis for Learning Disorders

Learning Disorders (i.e., Reading Disorder, Mathematics Disorder, Disorder of Written Expression) must be differentiated from . . .	In contrast to Learning Disorders, the other condition . . .
Normal variations in academic attainment	• Is not clinically significant or is not substantially below that expected given IQ and academic opportunities.
Lack of opportunity, poor teaching, cultural factors	• Results from factors external to the individual.
Poor academic performance due to impaired vision or hearing	• Is not in excess of what would be expected given the sensory deficit. A Learning Disorder can be diagnosed if the academic difficulties are in excess.
Mental Retardation	• Consists of an overall impairment in intellectual functioning that is not confined to a particular academic skill.
Pervasive Developmental Disorders	• Includes qualitative impairments in social skills and a restricted repertoire of interests or activities and is not confined to a particular academic skill.
Communication Disorders	• Is confined to impairment in speech or language skills (not academic skills).

Differential Diagnosis for Communication Disorders

Communication Disorders (i.e., Expressive Language, Mixed Receptive-Expressive Language, Phonological Disorders, and Stuttering) must be differentiated from . . .	In contrast to Communication Disorders, the other condition . . .
Mental Retardation	• Consists of an overall impairment in intellectual functioning as opposed to language impairment. A Communication Disorder can be diagnosed if the language problems are in excess of those usually associated with Mental Retardation.
Communication difficulties related to sensory or speech-motor deficits	• Is not in excess of that expected given the sensory or speech-motor deficit. A Communication Disorder can be diagnosed if the language problems are in excess of those usually associated with the deficits.
Normal dysfluencies or articulation difficulties in young children	• Is developmentally appropriate.

Differential Diagnosis for Autistic Disorder

Autistic Disorder must be differentiated from . . .	In contrast to Autistic Disorder, the other condition . . .
Rett's Disorder	• Occurs only in girls and includes characteristic features (e.g., deceleration in head growth, loss of hand movements, poor coordination).
Childhood Disintegrative Disorder	• Follows a period of at least 2 years of normal development and includes a loss of previously acquired skills.
Asperger's Disorder	• Does not have significant delay in language development.
Schizophrenia	• Has a later age at onset and includes characteristic features (e.g., delusions, hallucinations). In an individual with a history of Autistic Disorder or another Pervasive Developmental Disorder, Schizophrenia can be diagnosed only if there are prominent delusions or hallucinations.
Selective Mutism	• Is characterized by normal speech and social skills in certain situations.
Language Disorder	• Involves no qualitative impairment in social interaction, and the range of interests and behaviors is not restricted. A Language Disorder is not diagnosed if the criteria are met for a Pervasive Development Disorder.
Mental Retardation	• Involves general impairment in intellectual functioning; frequently accompanies Autistic Disorder.

(continued)

Differential Diagnosis for
Autistic Disorder *(continued)*

Autistic Disorder must be differentiated from . . .	In contrast to Autistic Disorder, the other condition . . .
Stereotypic Movement Disorder	• Occurs in the absence of impairment of social interaction and language development. Stereotypic Movement Disorder is not diagnosed if the stereotypy is part of a Pervasive Developmental Disorder.

Differential Diagnosis for
Attention-Deficit/Hyperactivity Disorder

Attention-Deficit/ Hyperactivity Disorder must be differentiated from . . .	In contrast to Attention-Deficit/ Hyperactivity Disorder, the other condition . . .
Age-appropriate behaviors in active children	• Does not cause clinically significant impairment.
Understimulating environments	• Leads to inattention that is related to boredom.
Inattention in Oppositional Defiant Disorder	• Results from unwillingness to conform to others' demands.
Impulsivity in Conduct Disorder	• Is associated with a pattern of antisocial behavior.
Inattention or hyperactivity associated with Pervasive Developmental Disorders	• Has a characteristic symptom presentation with marked defects in social relatedness, serious delays in language, and a restricted range of interests and behaviors.
Inattention or hyperactivity caused by drugs of abuse or medications (e.g., bronchodilator)	• Remits when drug of abuse or medication is discontinued and is diagnosed as Substance-Related Disorder Not Otherwise Specified or Adverse Effects of Medication Not Otherwise Specified.
Symptoms of inattention due to other mental disorders (e.g., Mood or Anxiety Disorders)	• Has the characteristic features of the other mental disorder, and onset is typically after age 7 years. Attention-Deficit/Hyperactivity Disorder is not diagnosed if inattention occurs exclusively during the course of a Pervasive Developmental Disorder, Schizophrenia, or other Psychotic Disorder, or if it is better accounted for by another mental disorder.

Differential Diagnosis for Conduct Disorder

Conduct Disorder must be differentiated from . . .	In contrast to Conduct Disorder, the other condition . . .
Disruptive behavior in Oppositional Defiant Disorder	• Focuses on negativistic and defiant symptoms that are less severe and not antisocial in nature. Oppositional Defiant Disorder is not diagnosed if criteria are met for Conduct Disorder.
Disruptive behavior in Attention-Deficit/Hyperactivity Disorder	• Focuses on hyperactive or impulse-control symptoms that are not antisocial in nature.
Antisocial behavior occurring during a Manic Episode	• Is accompanied by elevated or irritable mood (and other additional characteristic symptoms) and is more likely to occur only during circumscribed periods of disturbance.
Antisocial behavior related to a Psychotic Disorder	• Occurs only in response to delusions or hallucinations.
Adjustment Disorder	• Is below the severity threshold for Conduct Disorder and clearly occurs in response to a psychosocial stressor as opposed to being part of a long-standing pattern.
Child or Adolescent Antisocial Behavior	• Is below the severity threshold for Conduct Disorder or is not part of a long-standing pattern (i.e., isolated antisocial acts).
Antisocial Personality Disorder	• Can be diagnosed only in individuals over age 18 years. Conduct Disorder is not diagnosed if the individual is age 18 or older and if criteria are met for Antisocial Personality Disorder.

Differential Diagnosis for Oppositional Defiant Disorder

Oppositional Defiant Disorder must be differentiated from . . .	In contrast to Oppositional Defiant Disorder, the other condition . . .
Nonpathological oppositional behavior typical of certain developmental stages	• Is not clinically significant or is not a persistent pattern.
Adjustment Disorder With Disturbance of Conduct	• Is a maladaptive response to a stressor and does not meet criteria for Oppositional Defiant Disorder.
Conduct Disorder	• Is more severe and is characterized by aggressive and antisocial behaviors. Oppositional Defiant Disorder is not diagnosed if criteria are met for Conduct Disorder.
Oppositional behavior related to Mood or Psychotic Disorders	• Occurs only in the context of the mood disturbance or in relation to delusions or hallucinations.
Oppositional behavior related to Attention-Deficit/ Hyperactivity Disorder	• Occurs secondarily to frustration brought on by problems with inattention and hyperactivity.
Oppositional behavior in Mental Retardation	• Is less severe and is accompanied by a generalized delay in intellectual development.
Failure to follow directions due to impaired language comprehension	• Does not occur when communication is provided in the native language at a level the individual can understand.
Antisocial Personality Disorder	• Can be diagnosed only in individuals over age 18 years.

Differential Diagnosis for Tic Disorders

Tic Disorders (e.g., Tourette's Disorder) must be differentiated from . . .	In contrast to Tic Disorders, the other condition . . .
Abnormal movements associated with general medical conditions	• Is due to the direct physiological effects of a general medical condition.
Tics caused by drugs of abuse or medications (e.g., stimulants)	• Remits when drug of abuse or medication is discontinued and is diagnosed as Substance-Related Disorder Not Otherwise Specified or Medication-Induced Movement Disorder Not Otherwise Specified.
Stereotypic Movement Disorder, Stereotypies in Pervasive Developmental Disorders	• Is characterized by nonfunctional, usually rhythmic, seemingly driven behaviors that are generally more complex than tics.
Compulsions in Obsessive-Compulsive Disorder	• Occurs in response to an obsession or according to rigidly applied rules.
Disorganized or bizarre vocalizations or behaviors in Schizophrenia	• Is accompanied by the other characteristic symptoms (e.g., delusions, negative symptoms) and course (e.g., marked decline in functioning).

Differential Diagnosis for
Separation Anxiety Disorder

Separation Anxiety Disorder must be differentiated from . . .	In contrast to Separation Anxiety Disorder, the other condition . . .
School refusal in Social Phobia	• Is due to fear of embarrassment in school rather than fears of separation from home.
Pervasive Developmental Disorders	• Is characterized by marked impairment in social relatedness that occurs in all relationships, including those with close family members. Separation Anxiety Disorder is not diagnosed if the behavior occurs exclusively during the course of a Pervasive Developmental Disorder.
Psychotic Disorders	• Has a later age at onset, and the social awkwardness is related to delusional fears or negative symptoms. Separation Anxiety Disorder is not diagnosed if the behavior occurs exclusively during the course of Schizophrenia or another Psychotic Disorder.
Generalized Anxiety Disorder	• Is characterized by anxiety and worry in a multitude of different areas and is not limited to issues of separation from family.
Panic Disorder With Agoraphobia, Agoraphobia Without History of Panic Disorder	• Has a later age at onset, and the focus of the fear, anxiety, and avoidance is on situations in which a Panic Attack (or incapacitating symptoms) might occur. In adolescents and adults, Separation Anxiety Disorder is not diagnosed if the disturbance is better accounted for by Panic Disorder With Agoraphobia.

(continued)

Differential Diagnosis for
Separation Anxiety Disorder *(continued)*

Separation Anxiety Disorder must be differentiated from . . .	In contrast to Separation Anxiety Disorder, the other condition . . .
Truancy in Conduct Disorder	• Is not related to the inability to separate from attachment figures and is associated with other conduct symptoms.
School refusal in Mood Disorders	• Is due to loss of interest, fatigue, or concern about crying in public.
Developmentally appropriate levels of anxiety	• Is not clinically significant.

Delirium, Dementia, Amnestic Disorder

Differential Diagnosis for Delirium

Delirium (characterized by clouding of consciousness) must be differentiated from . . .	In contrast to Delirium, the other condition . . .
Cognitive deficits in Dementia	• Is characterized by a relatively stable or gradually progressive course; typically is of a much longer duration; and, although characterized by a number of cognitive deficits, the ability to maintain attention is not impaired. Episodes of Delirium can occur in a preexisting Dementia. Dementia is not diagnosed if the deficits occur exclusively during the course of Delirium. When Delirium occurs in the context of a preexisting Dementia, it should be separately diagnosed.
Disturbance in consciousness in Substance Intoxication or Substance Withdrawal	• Is *not* in excess of that usually associated with the characteristic intoxication or withdrawal syndrome or is not severe enough to warrant independent clinical attention. Substance-Induced Delirium is diagnosed instead of Substance Intoxication or Withdrawal only when the disturbance is in excess of what is expected and when it is severe enough to warrant independent attention.

(continued)

Differential Diagnosis for Delirium *(continued)*

Delirium (characterized by clouding of consciousness) must be differentiated from . . .	In contrast to Delirium, the other condition . . .
Hallucinations or delusions in Substance-Induced Psychotic Disorder or Psychotic Disorder Due to a General Medical Condition	• Is not accompanied by a disturbance in consciousness and other cognitive deficits characteristic of Delirium. Substance-Induced Psychotic Disorder and Psychotic Disorder Due to a General Medical Condition are not diagnosed if the psychotic symptoms occur exclusively during Delirium.
Hallucinations or delusions in Psychotic Disorders or Mood Disorders With Psychotic Features	• Is not due to the direct effects of a general medical condition or substance use.
Agitation in Manic or Major Depressive Episode or Psychotic Disorder	• Is not due to the direct effects of a general medical condition or substance use.

Differential Diagnosis for Dementia

Dementia (memory and other cognitive impairments) must be differentiated from . . .	In contrast to Dementia, the other condition . . .
Delirium	• Is characterized by a disturbance in consciousness and a fluctuating course. Dementia is not diagnosed if the cognitive deficits occur exclusively during Delirium. However, periods of Delirium can occur in the context of a Dementia and should be diagnosed if present.
Amnestic Disorder	• Is characterized by memory impairment occurring in the absence of other cognitive deficits (i.e., aphasia, agnosia, apraxia, executive functioning). Amnestic Disorder is not diagnosed if the memory disturbance occurs exclusively during Dementia.
Cognitive impairment in Substance Intoxication or Substance Withdrawal	• Remits when the acute effects of intoxication or withdrawal subside. In contrast, Substance-Induced Persisting Dementia may be diagnosed if the Dementia persists long beyond the period of intoxication or withdrawal.
Mental Retardation	• Must have an onset before age 18 years.
Cognitive impairment and deterioration in functioning in Schizophrenia	• Has a generally earlier age at onset, less severe cognitive impairment, a characteristic symptom pattern (e.g., delusions and hallucinations), and is not due to the direct effects of a general medical condition or substance use.

(continued)

Differential Diagnosis for Dementia *(continued)*

Dementia (memory and other cognitive impairments) must be differentiated from . . .	In contrast to Dementia, the other condition . . .
Memory deficits and difficulty concentrating in Major Depressive Disorder	• Improves when the depression remits, is associated with other characteristic depressive symptoms, is often associated with prior history (or family history) of depression, and is not due to the direct effects of a general medical condition or substance use.
Age-Related Cognitive Decline	• Is characterized by cognitive impairment that is in keeping with what would be expected for the individual's age and is not due to the direct effects of a general medical condition or substance use.
Mild Neurocognitive Disorder (i.e., Cognitive Disorder Not Otherwise Specified)	• Does not meet the severity threshold for Dementia.

Differential Diagnosis for Amnestic Disorder

Amnestic Disorder must be differentiated from . . .	In contrast to Amnestic Disorder, the other condition . . .
Delirium	• Is characterized by a disturbance in consciousness and a fluctuating course. Amnestic Disorder cannot be diagnosed if the memory disturbance occurs exclusively during the course of Delirium.
Dementia	• Is characterized by the presence of cognitive deficits (i.e., agnosia, aphasia, apraxia, executive functioning) in addition to memory disturbance. Amnestic Disorder cannot be diagnosed if the memory disturbance occurs exclusively during the course of Delirium.
Dissociative Amnesia, amnesia occurring in other Dissociative Disorders	• Usually involves a circumscribed loss of memory related to traumatic events and is not due to the direct effects of a general medical condition or substance use.
Memory impairment in Substance Intoxication or Substance Withdrawal	• Remits when the acute effects of intoxication or withdrawal subside. In contrast, Substance-Induced Persisting Amnestic Disorder may be diagnosed if the memory impairment persists long beyond the period of intoxication or withdrawal.
Memory deficits in Major Depressive Disorder	• Improves when the depression remits, is often associated with prior history (or family history) of depression, and is not due to the direct effects of a general medical condition or substance use.

(continued)

Differential Diagnosis for
Amnestic Disorder *(continued)*

Amnestic Disorder must be differentiated from . . .	In contrast to Amnestic Disorder, the other condition . . .
Malingering, Factitious Disorder	• Is characterized by the feigning of lost memories.
Age-Related Cognitive Decline	• Is characterized by memory impairment that is in keeping with what would be expected for the individual's age and is not due to the direct effects of a general medical condition or substance use.

Mental Disorders Due to a General Medical Condition

Differential Diagnosis for Catatonic Disorder Due to a General Medical Condition

Catatonic Disorder Due to a General Medical Condition must be differentiated from . . .	In contrast to Catatonic Disorder Due to a General Medical Condition, the other condition . . .
Mutism or posturing in Delirium	• Is characterized by a clouding of consciousness and other cognitive deficits. Catatonic Disorder is not diagnosed if the symptoms occur exclusively during the course of Delirium.
Akinesia, rigidity, or posturing in Medication-Induced Movement Disorders	• Is due to the direct physiological effects of a medication.
Schizophrenia, Catatonic Type	• Is not due to the direct effects of a general medical condition and is accompanied by other characteristic symptoms of Schizophrenia.
Mood Disorder With Catatonic Features	• Is not due to the direct effects of a general medical condition and is accompanied by other characteristic symptoms of Mood Disorder.

Differential Diagnosis for Personality Change Due to a General Medical Condition

Personality Change Due to a General Medical Condition must be differentiated from . . .	In contrast to Personality Change Due to a General Medical Condition, the other condition . . .
Personality Change as an associated feature in Delirium	• Includes fluctuating cognitive deficits in addition to personality changes. Personality Change is not diagnosed if the personality disturbance occurs exclusively during the course of Delirium.
Personality Change as an associated feature in Dementia	• Includes memory impairment and other cognitive deficits in addition to personality changes. Personality Change Due to a General Medical Condition may be diagnosed in addition to the Dementia if the personality disturbance is a prominent feature.
Personality Change associated with another Mental Disorder Due to a General Medical Condition (e.g., Mood Disorder Due to a General Medical Condition)	• Includes additional features (e.g., depressed mood). Personality Change is not diagnosed if the disturbance is better accounted for by another Mental Disorder Due to a General Medical Condition.
Personality Change as a result of Substance Dependence	• Is not due to the direct effects of a general medical condition and remits when the dependence is in remission.
Personality Change associated with another mental disorder (e.g., Delusional Disorder)	• Is not due to the direct effects of a general medical condition.
Personality Disorder	• Has a different age at onset, course, and characteristic features and is not due to the direct effects of a general medical condition.

Schizophrenia and Other Psychotic Disorders

Differential Diagnosis for Schizophrenia

Schizophrenia must be differentiated from . . .	In contrast to Schizophrenia, the other condition . . .
Psychotic Disorder Due to a General Medical Condition, Delirium, Dementia	• Requires the presence of an etiological general medical condition. Schizophrenia is not diagnosed if the psychotic symptoms are all due to the direct physiological effects of a general medical condition.
Substance-Induced Psychotic Disorder, Substance-Induced Delirium	• Requires that the psychotic symptoms be initiated and maintained by substance use (including medication side effects). Schizophrenia is not diagnosed if the psychotic symptoms are all due to the direct physiological effects of a substance (including medication).
Schizoaffective Disorder	• Is characterized by mood symptoms that are present for a substantial portion of the total duration of the active and residual periods of the illness (as opposed to Schizophrenia, in which the mood symptoms are brief relative to the total duration).
Mood Disorder With Psychotic Features	• Is characterized by psychotic symptoms that occur exclusively during periods of mood disturbance.
Schizophreniform Disorder	• Is characterized by a total duration between 1 and 6 months.
Brief Psychotic Disorder	• Is characterized by a total duration of less than 1 month.

(continued)

Differential Diagnosis for
Schizophrenia *(continued)*

Schizophrenia must be differentiated from . . .	In contrast to Schizophrenia, the other condition . . .
Delusional Disorder	• Is characterized by nonbizarre delusions occurring in the absence of other clinically significant psychotic symptoms (including negative symptoms).
Pervasive Developmental Disorders	• Is characterized by an early onset (e.g., before age 3 for Autistic Disorder) and an absence of prominent delusions or hallucinations. A diagnosis of Schizophrenia is warranted in individuals with a preexisting diagnosis of Autistic Disorder only if prominent hallucinations or delusions have been present for at least a month.
Schizotypal, Schizoid, or Paranoid Personality Disorder	• Is not characterized by psychotic symptoms. An additional diagnosis of Schizophrenia is appropriate when the symptoms are severe enough to satisfy Criterion A of Schizophrenia. In such cases, the preexisting Personality Disorder may be noted on Axis II followed by "(premorbid)."

Differential Diagnosis for Schizoaffective Disorder

Schizoaffective Disorder must be differentiated from . . .	In contrast to Schizoaffective Disorder, the other condition . . .
Psychotic Disorder Due to a General Medical Condition, Delirium, Dementia	• Requires the presence of an etiological general medical condition. Schizoaffective Disorder is not diagnosed if the psychotic or mood symptoms are all due to the direct physiological effects of a general medical condition.
Substance-Induced Psychotic Disorder, Substance-Induced Delirium	• Requires that the psychotic and mood symptoms be initiated and maintained by substance use (including medication side effects). Schizoaffective Disorder is not diagnosed if the psychotic or mood symptoms are all due to the direct physiological effects of a substance (including medication).
Schizophrenia	• Is characterized by mood symptoms that are brief relative to the total duration of the illness.
Mood Disorder With Psychotic Features	• Is characterized by psychotic symptoms that occur exclusively during mood episodes.
Delusional Disorder	• Is characterized by nonbizarre delusions occurring in the absence of other symptoms that meet Criterion A of Schizophrenia.

Differential Diagnosis for Delusional Disorder

Delusional Disorder must be differentiated from . . .	In contrast to Delusional Disorder, the other condition . . .
Delirium, Dementia, Psychotic Disorder Due to a General Medical Condition	• Requires the presence of an etiological general medical condition. Delusional Disorder is not diagnosed if the delusions are all due to the direct physiological effects of a general medical condition.
Substance-Induced Psychotic Disorder	• Requires that the psychotic symptoms be initiated and maintained by substance use (including medication side effects). Delusional Disorder is not diagnosed if the delusions are all due to the direct physiological effects of a substance (including medication).
Schizophrenia, Schizophreniform Disorder	• Is characterized by the presence of other symptoms (in addition to prominent delusions) that meet Criterion A for Schizophrenia.
Mood Disorder With Psychotic Features	• Is characterized by delusions that occur exclusively during the mood episodes.
Shared Psychotic Disorder	• Is characterized by delusions that arise only in the context of a close relationship with a dominant person who has delusions.
Brief Psychotic Disorder	• Is characterized by psychotic symptoms that last for less than 1 month.
Hypochondriasis, Obsessive-Compulsive Disorder, Body Dysmorphic Disorder	• Is characterized by excessive, unrealistic, and distorted overvalued ideas that are generally held with less than delusional conviction.

(continued)

Differential Diagnosis for
Delusional Disorder *(continued)*

Delusional Disorder must be differentiated from . . .	In contrast to Delusional Disorder, the other condition . . .
Paranoid Personality Disorder	• Is characterized by paranoid ideation without clear-cut or persisting delusional beliefs. When a person with a Delusional Disorder has a preexisting Paranoid Personality Disorder, the Personality Disorder should be listed on Axis II followed by "(premorbid)."

Differential Diagnosis for Brief Psychotic Disorder

Brief Psychotic Disorder must be differentiated from . . .	In contrast to Brief Psychotic Disorder, the other condition . . .
Psychotic Disorder Due to a General Medical Condition, Delirium	• Requires the presence of an etiological general medical condition. Brief Psychotic Disorder is not diagnosed if the psychotic symptoms are all due to the direct physiological effects of a general medical condition.
Substance-Induced Psychotic Disorder, Substance-Induced Delirium, Substance Intoxication, Substance Withdrawal	• Requires that the psychotic symptoms be initiated and maintained by substance use (including medication side effects). Brief Psychotic Disorder is not diagnosed if the psychotic symptoms are all due to the direct physiological effects of a substance (including medication).
Mood Disorders With Psychotic Features	• Is characterized by psychotic symptoms occurring exclusively during mood episodes. Brief Psychotic Disorder is not diagnosed if the psychotic symptoms are better accounted for by a Mood Disorder.
Schizophreniform Disorder, Schizophrenia, Delusional Disorder	• Is characterized by psychotic symptoms that last for 1 month or longer.
Psychotic symptoms occurring in the context of some Personality Disorders (e.g., Borderline)	• Are usually transient and lasts less than 1 day. If clinically significant, they may be diagnosed as Psychotic Disorder Not Otherwise Specified. If psychotic symptoms persist for at least 1 day, the additional diagnosis of Brief Psychotic Disorder may be warranted.

Mood Disorders

Differential Diagnosis for Major Depressive Disorder

Major Depressive Disorder must be differentiated from . . .	In contrast to Major Depressive Disorder, the other condition . . .
Bipolar I or Bipolar II Disorder	• Includes one or more Manic, Mixed, or Hypomanic Episodes. Major Depressive Disorder cannot be diagnosed if a Manic, Mixed, or Hypomanic Episode has ever been present.
Mood Disorder Due to a General Medical Condition	• Requires the presence of an etiological general medical condition. Major Depressive Disorder is not diagnosed if the major depressive-like episodes are all due to the direct physiological effects of a general medical condition.
Substance-Induced Mood Disorder	• Is due to the direct physiological effects of a substance. Major Depressive Disorder is not diagnosed if the major depressive-like episodes are all due to the direct physiological effects of a substance (including medication).
Dysthymic Disorder	• Is characterized by depressed mood, more days than not, for at least 2 years and the absence of Major Depressive Episodes during the first 2 years of the dysthymic disturbance. Both can be diagnosed if the Major Depressive Episodes have their onset after at least 2 years of Dysthymic Disorder.

(continued)

Differential Diagnosis for
Major Depressive Disorder *(continued)*

Major Depressive Disorder must be differentiated from . . .	In contrast to Major Depressive Disorder, the other condition . . .
Schizoaffective Disorder	• Is characterized by a period of at least 2 weeks of delusions or hallucinations occurring in the absence of prominent mood symptoms.
Schizophrenia, Delusional Disorder, Psychotic Disorder Not Otherwise Specified	• May include mood symptoms that are brief relative to the total duration of the psychotic disturbance. Major Depressive Episodes superimposed on a Psychotic Disorder should be diagnosed as Depressive Disorder Not Otherwise Specified.
Dementia	• Is characterized by a premorbid history of declining cognitive functioning.
Adjustment Disorder With Depressed Mood	• Is characterized by depressive symptoms that occur in response to a stressor and do not meet criteria for a Major Depressive Episode.
Bereavement	• Occurs in response to the loss of a loved one and is generally less severe than a Major Depressive Episode. When the full symptom picture of a Major Depressive Episode occurs after the loss of a loved one, it persists for less than 2 months after the loss and is not characterized by marked functional impairment, morbid preoccupation with worthlessness, suicidal ideation, psychotic symptoms, or psychomotor retardation.

(continued)

Differential Diagnosis for
Major Depressive Disorder *(continued)*

Major Depressive Disorder must be differentiated from . . .	In contrast to Major Depressive Disorder, the other condition . . .
Nonpathological periods of sadness	• Is characterized by short duration, few associated symptoms, and lack of significant functional impairment or distress.

Differential Diagnosis for Dysthymic Disorder

Dysthymic Disorder must be differentiated from . . .	In contrast to Dysthymic Disorder, the other condition . . .
Major Depressive Disorder	• Is characterized by one or more Major Depressive Episodes. Both Dysthymic Disorder and Major Depressive Disorder can be diagnosed if the Major Depressive Episodes have their onset after the first 2 years of the Dysthymic Disorder.
Depressive symptoms associated with chronic Psychotic Disorders	• Occurs exclusively during the psychotic disturbance. Dysthymic Disorder is not diagnosed if the depressive symptoms occur exclusively during a chronic Psychotic Disorder.
Mood Disorder Due to a General Medical Condition	• Requires the presence of an etiological general medical condition. Dysthymic Disorder is not diagnosed if the depressive symptoms are all due to the direct physiological effects of a general medical condition.
Substance-Induced Mood Disorder	• Is due to the direct physiological effects of a substance. Dysthymic Disorder is not diagnosed if depressive symptoms are all due to the direct physiological effects of a substance (including medication).
Cyclothymic Disorder	• Is characterized by hypomanic periods in addition to depressive periods. Dysthymic Disorder cannot be diagnosed if the criteria have ever been met for Cyclothymic Disorder.
Nonpathological periods of sadness	• Is characterized by short duration, few associated symptoms, and lack of significant functional impairment or distress.

Differential Diagnosis for Bipolar I Disorder

Bipolar I Disorder must be differentiated from . . .	In contrast to Bipolar I Disorder, the other condition . . .
Mood Disorder Due to a General Medical Condition	• Requires the presence of an etiological general medical condition. Bipolar I Disorder is not diagnosed if the mood episodes are all due to the direct physiological effects of a general medical condition.
Substance-Induced Mood Disorder	• Is due to the direct physiological effects of a substance. Bipolar I Disorder is not diagnosed if the mood episodes are all due to the direct physiological effects of a substance (including antidepressant medication).
Major Depressive Disorder, Dysthymic Disorder	• Is characterized by the absence of Manic Episodes. Major Depressive Disorder and Dysthymic Disorder are not diagnosed if there has ever been a Manic, Mixed, or unequivocal Hypomanic Episode.
Bipolar II Disorder	• Is characterized by the presence of Hypomanic and Major Depressive Episodes and the absence of Manic or Mixed Episodes. Bipolar II Disorder cannot be diagnosed if the criteria have ever been met for Bipolar I Disorder.

(continued)

Differential Diagnosis for Bipolar I Disorder *(continued)*

Bipolar I Disorder must be differentiated from . . .	In contrast to Bipolar I Disorder, the other condition . . .
Cyclothymic Disorder	• Is characterized by numerous periods of hypomanic symptoms that do not meet criteria for a Manic Episode and periods of depressive symptoms that do not meet criteria for a Major Depressive Episode. Both Bipolar I Disorder and Cyclothymic Disorder can be diagnosed if the Manic or Mixed Episodes occur after at least 2 years of Cyclothymic Disorder.
Psychotic Disorders (nonmood)	• Is characterized by periods of psychotic symptoms that occur in the absence of prominent mood symptoms. Bipolar Disorder Not Otherwise Specified is diagnosed for Manic Episodes superimposed on a chronic Psychotic Disorder.

Differential Diagnosis for Bipolar II Disorder

Bipolar II Disorder must be differentiated from . . .	In contrast to Bipolar II Disorder, the other condition . . .
Mood Disorder Due to a General Medical Condition	• Requires the presence of an etiological general medical condition. Bipolar II Disorder is not diagnosed if the mood episodes are all due to the direct physiological effects of a general medical condition.
Substance-Induced Mood Disorder	• Is due to the direct physiological effects of a substance. Bipolar II Disorder is not diagnosed if the mood episodes are all due to the direct physiological effects of a substance (including antidepressant medication).
Major Depressive Disorder, Dysthymic Disorder	• Is characterized by the absence of unequivocal Hypomanic Episodes. Major Depressive Disorder and Dysthymic Disorder cannot be diagnosed if the criteria have ever been met for Bipolar II Disorder.
Bipolar I Disorder	• Is characterized by the presence of at least one Manic or Mixed Episode. Bipolar II Disorder cannot be diagnosed if the criteria have ever been met for Bipolar I Disorder.
Cyclothymic Disorder	• Is characterized by numerous periods of depressive symptoms, but none of these meet criteria for a Major Depressive Episode. Both Bipolar II Disorder and Cyclothymic Disorder can be diagnosed if Major Depressive Episodes occur after at least 2 years of Cyclothymic Disorder.

(continued)

Differential Diagnosis for Bipolar II Disorder *(continued)*

Bipolar II Disorder must be differentiated from . . .	In contrast to Bipolar II Disorder, the other condition . . .
Psychotic Disorders (nonmood)	• Is characterized by periods of psychotic symptoms that occur in the absence of prominent mood symptoms.

Differential Diagnosis for Cyclothymic Disorder

Cyclothymic Disorder must be differentiated from . . .	In contrast to Cyclothymic Disorder, the other condition . . .
Bipolar I or Bipolar II Disorder, With Rapid Cycling	• Is characterized by four or more mood episodes (each of which meets full criteria for a Manic, Mixed, Hypomanic, or Major Depressive Episode) occurring in a 12-month period.
Borderline Personality Disorder	• Is characterized by additional personality features (e.g., identity disturbance, self-mutilating behavior) besides affective lability.
Mood Disorder Due to a General Medical Condition	• Requires the presence of an etiological general medical condition. Cyclothymic Disorder is not diagnosed if the mood symptoms are all due to the direct physiological effects of a general medical condition.
Substance-Induced Mood Disorder	• Is due to the direct physiological effects of a substance. Cyclothymic Disorder is not diagnosed if the mood symptoms are all due to the direct physiological effects of a substance (including medication).

Anxiety Disorders

Differential Diagnosis for
Panic Disorder With Agoraphobia

Panic Disorder With Agoraphobia must be differentiated from . . .	In contrast to Panic Disorder With Agoraphobia, the other condition . . .
Anxiety Disorder Due to a General Medical Condition	• Requires the presence of an etiological general medical condition. Panic Disorder is not diagnosed if the Panic Attacks are all due to the direct physiological effects of a general medical condition.
Substance-Induced Anxiety Disorder	• Is due to the direct physiological effects of a substance. Panic Disorder is not diagnosed if the Panic Attacks are all due to the direct physiological effects of a substance (including medication).
Panic Attacks occurring as part of another Anxiety Disorder (e.g., Social Phobia, Specific Phobia, Obsessive-Compulsive Disorder, Posttraumatic Stress Disorder)	• Is characterized by Panic Attacks that are either situationally bound or situationally predisposed (as opposed to the unexpected Panic Attacks, which are required in Panic Disorder).
Separation Anxiety Disorder	• Must have its onset in childhood and is characterized by anxiety and avoidance that is focused on separation concerns.
Avoidance in Delusional Disorder	• Results from delusional concerns.

Differential Diagnosis for Agoraphobia Without History of Panic Disorder

Agoraphobia Without History of Panic Disorder must be differentiated from . . .	In contrast to Agoraphobia Without History of Panic Disorder, the other condition . . .
Panic Disorder With Agoraphobia	• Is characterized by recurrent unexpected Panic Attacks preceding the onset of the Agoraphobia.
Social Phobia	• Is characterized by avoidance of performance in social situations in which the person will be exposed to the scrutiny of others.
Specific Phobia	• Is characterized by avoidance of a specific feared object or situation, which, at least initially, is not related to concerns about being unable to escape in the event of developing paniclike symptoms.
Being housebound in Major Depressive Disorder	• May result from feelings of apathy, fatigue, loss of capacity to experience pleasure, or concerns about crying in public.
Avoidance in Delusional Disorder	• Results from delusional concerns (e.g., of being followed).
Avoidance in Obsessive-Compulsive Disorder	• Is intended to prevent triggering an obsession or compulsion (e.g., avoidance of "dirty" objects related to fears of contamination or avoidance of objects that might be used as weapons in someone who is having obsessive fears of harming someone).
Separation Anxiety Disorder	• Is characterized by avoidance of situations that involve being away from home or close relatives.

(continued)

Differential Diagnosis for Agoraphobia Without History of Panic Disorder *(continued)*

Agoraphobia Without History of Panic Disorder must be differentiated from . . .	In contrast to Agoraphobia Without History of Panic Disorder, the other condition . . .
Avoidance that results from realistic concerns associated with a general medical condition (e.g., fainting in an individual with an arrhythmia)	• Is at a level that is appropriate given the nature of the general medical condition.

Differential Diagnosis for Specific Phobia

Specific Phobia must be differentiated from . . .	In contrast to Specific Phobia, the other condition . . .
Panic Disorder With Agoraphobia	• Is characterized by recurrent unexpected Panic Attacks and avoidance of typically many different situations.
Social Phobia	• Is characterized by fear and avoidance of social situations.
Avoidance in Posttraumatic Stress Disorder	• Is related to stimuli that remind the individual of a previously experienced life-threatening event.
Avoidance in Obsessive-Compulsive Disorder	• Is associated with the content of the obsessions (e.g., dirt, contamination).
Avoidance in Separation Anxiety Disorder	• Is associated with fear of separation from parents or caretakers.
Avoidance in Psychotic Disorders	• Is in response to a delusion (without the recognition that the fear is excessive or unreasonable).
Nonpathological avoidance of circumscribed objects or situations	• Lacks clinically significant impairment or distress (e.g., person who fears snakes but lives in Manhattan).

Differential Diagnosis for Social Phobia

Social Phobia must be differentiated from . . .	In contrast to Social Phobia, the other condition . . .
Panic Disorder With Agoraphobia	• Is typically not limited to social situations and is characterized by the initial onset of unexpected Panic Attacks.
Agoraphobia Without History of Panic Disorder, Generalized Anxiety Disorder, Specific Phobia	• Involves anxiety or avoidance that is not limited to situations that involve scrutiny by others.
Separation Anxiety Disorder	• Is characterized by fears concerning separation from caretakers.
Pervasive Developmental Disorders, Schizoid Personality Disorder	• Is characterized by avoidance of social situations due to a lack of interest in relating to other individuals.
Avoidant Personality Disorder	• Is conceptualized as a Personality Disorder but may describe the same group of patients as Social Phobia, Generalized Type. For individuals with Social Phobia, Generalized Type, an additional diagnosis of Avoidant Personality Disorder should be considered.
Social anxiety and avoidance associated with other mental disorders	• Is characterized by anxiety that occurs only during the course of the other mental disorder. If the anxiety is judged to be better accounted for by the other mental disorder, an additional diagnosis of Social Phobia is not given.
Nonpathological performance anxiety, stage fright, or shyness	• Lacks clinically significant impairment or marked distress.

Differential Diagnosis for Obsessive-Compulsive Disorder

Obsessive-Compulsive Disorder must be differentiated from . . .	In contrast to Obsessive-Compulsive Disorder, the other condition . . .
Anxiety Disorder Due to a General Medical Condition	• Requires the presence of an etiological general medical condition. Obsessive-Compulsive Disorder is not diagnosed if the obsessions and compulsions are all due to the direct physiological effects of a general medical condition.
Substance-Induced Anxiety Disorder	• Is due to the direct physiological effects of a substance. Obsessive-Compulsive Disorder is not diagnosed if the obsessions and compulsions are all due to the direct physiological effects of a substance (including medication).
Body Dysmorphic Disorder or Eating Disorder	• Is characterized by recurrent thoughts exclusively related to a preoccupation with appearance or body weight.
Specific or Social Phobia	• Is characterized by recurrent thoughts exclusively related to fear or avoidance of a feared object or situation.
Trichotillomania	• Is characterized by recurrent thoughts and actions related to hair pulling.
Hypochondriasis	• Is characterized by recurrent thoughts exclusively related to the idea that one has a serious disease.
Major Depressive Episode	• Is characterized by egosyntonic brooding and ruminations.

(continued)

Differential Diagnosis for Obsessive-Compulsive Disorder
(continued)

Obsessive-Compulsive Disorder must be differentiated from . . .	In contrast to Obsessive-Compulsive Disorder, the other condition . . .
Generalized Anxiety Disorder	• Is characterized by excessive concerns about realistic situations and is not accompanied by compulsions.
Delusional Disorder or Psychotic Disorder Not Otherwise Specified	• Is characterized by recurrent thoughts that are held with delusional conviction.
Schizophrenia	• Is characterized by ruminative delusional thoughts and stereotyped behaviors that are not subject to reality testing.
Tic or Stereotypic Movement Disorder	• Is characterized by movements that are less complex and are not aimed at neutralizing an obsession.
Driven behaviors associated with other mental disorders (e.g., Pathological Gambling, Paraphilias, Substance Dependence)	• Is characterized by the person's deriving pleasure from the activity and wanting to resist it only because of its deleterious consequences.
Obsessive-Compulsive Personality Disorder	• Is not characterized by the presence of obsessions or compulsions and involves a pervasive pattern of orderliness, perfectionism, and control.
Nonpathological superstitions and repetitive behaviors	• Is not time consuming and does not result in clinically significant impairment or distress.

Differential Diagnosis for Posttraumatic Stress Disorder

Posttraumatic Stress Disorder must be differentiated from . . .	In contrast to Posttraumatic Stress Disorder, the other condition . . .
Adjustment Disorder	• Is characterized by a stressor of any level of severity and does not have a specific response pattern (e.g., reexperiencing the trauma).
Other mental disorders that may occur after exposure to an extreme stressor	• Is characterized by a response pattern that meets criteria for another mental disorder (e.g., Brief Psychotic Disorder, Major Depressive Disorder).
Acute Stress Disorder	• Is characterized by a response pattern that occurs within 4 weeks of the stressor. If the symptoms persist for more than 1 month and meet criteria for Posttraumatic Stress Disorder, the diagnosis is changed from Acute Stress Disorder to Posttraumatic Stress Disorder.
Intrusive thoughts in Obsessive-Compulsive Disorder	• Is not related to an extreme stressor.
Malingering	• Is characterized by feigning of symptoms and should be ruled out when legal, financial, and other benefits play a role.

Differential Diagnosis for Acute Stress Disorder

Acute Stress Disorder must be differentiated from . . .	In contrast to Acute Stress Disorder, the other condition . . .
Mental Disorder Due to a General Medical Condition	• Requires the presence of an etiological general medical condition. Acute Stress Disorder is not diagnosed if the symptoms are all due to the physical effects of the stressful event (e.g., head injury).
Substance-Induced Disorder	• Is due to the direct physiological effects of a substance. Acute Stress Disorder is not diagnosed if the symptoms are due to the direct physiological effects of a substance (e.g., Alcohol Intoxication).
Brief Psychotic Disorder	• Is characterized by psychotic symptoms occurring in response to a stressor. In such cases, Brief Psychotic Disorder With Marked Stressors is diagnosed instead of Acute Stress Disorder.
Exacerbation of a preexisting mental disorder that was present before the exposure	• Has no additional symptoms after the stressor. A separate diagnosis of Acute Stress Disorder is not given.
Posttraumatic Stress Disorder	• Is characterized by symptoms lasting more than 1 month. If the symptoms of Acute Stress Disorder persist for more than 1 month, the diagnosis is changed to Posttraumatic Stress Disorder.
Adjustment Disorder	• Is characterized by a symptom pattern that does not meet criteria for any specific mental disorder (including Acute Stress Disorder).

(continued)

Differential Diagnosis for
Acute Stress Disorder *(continued)*

Acute Stress Disorder must be differentiated from . . .	In contrast to Acute Stress Disorder, the other condition . . .
Malingering	• Is characterized by feigning of symptoms and should be ruled out when legal, financial, and other benefits play a role.

Differential Diagnosis for Generalized Anxiety Disorder

Generalized Anxiety Disorder must be differentiated from . . .	In contrast to Generalized Anxiety Disorder, the other condition . . .
Anxiety Disorder Due to a General Medical Condition	• Requires the presence of an etiological general medical condition. Generalized Anxiety Disorder is not diagnosed if the generalized anxiety is due to the direct physiological effects of a general medical condition.
Substance-Induced Anxiety Disorder	• Is due to the direct physiological effects of a substance. Generalized Anxiety Disorder is not diagnosed if the generalized anxiety is due to the direct physiological effects of a substance (including medication).
Anxiety associated with another disorder (e.g., Hypochondriasis, Social Phobia)	• Is characterized by excessive anxiety and worry that is focused exclusively on the symptoms of the other disorder (e.g., anxiety related to fear of having a serious illness in Hypochondriasis). An additional diagnosis of Generalized Anxiety Disorder should be made only when the focus of the worry is unrelated to the other disorder.
Obsessions in Obsessive-Compulsive Disorder	• Is characterized by egodystonic intrusive thoughts that are usually accompanied by compulsions.
Posttraumatic Stress Disorder	• Is characterized by anxiety that is associated with reexperiencing a traumatic event. Generalized Anxiety Disorder is not diagnosed if the anxiety occurs exclusively during the course of Posttraumatic Stress Disorder.

(continued)

Differential Diagnosis for
Generalized Anxiety Disorder
(continued)

Generalized Anxiety Disorder must be differentiated from . . .	In contrast to Generalized Anxiety Disorder, the other condition . . .
Adjustment Disorder With Anxiety	• Does not meet the criteria for any specific Anxiety Disorder (including Generalized Anxiety Disorder) and must occur in response to a stressor.
Mood Disorders, Psychotic Disorders	• May be characterized by anxiety as an associated feature but includes other specific symptoms. Generalized Anxiety Disorder should not be diagnosed separately if it occurs exclusively during the course of a Mood or Psychotic Disorder.
Nonpathological anxiety	• Is characterized by worries that are more controllable and realistic.

Somatoform Disorders

Differential Diagnosis for Somatization Disorder

Somatization Disorder must be differentiated from . . .	In contrast to Somatization Disorder, the other condition . . .
General medical condition	• Fully accounts for the physical complaints.
Undifferentiated Somatoform Disorder	• Requires fewer symptoms and a shorter minimum duration (6 months versus several years). Undifferentiated Somatoform Disorder is not diagnosed if the symptoms are better accounted for by Somatization Disorder.
Pain Disorder, Sexual Dysfunction, Conversion Disorder, Dissociative Disorder	• Does not have multiple somatic complaints affecting a variety of organ systems and sites. None of these disorders are diagnosed if the symptoms occur exclusively during the course of Somatization Disorder.
Generalized Anxiety Disorder	• Is characterized by worry not limited to physical complaints.
Panic Disorder	• Has somatic complaints occurring only during Panic Attacks.
Depressive Disorders	• May have somatic complaints that are limited to episodes of depressed mood.
Schizophrenia or other Psychotic Disorders	• May have somatic concerns that are of a delusional nature.

(continued)

Differential Diagnosis for
Somatization Disorder *(continued)*

Somatization Disorder must be differentiated from . . .	In contrast to Somatization Disorder, the other condition . . .
Factitious Disorder, Malingering	• Is characterized by symptoms that are intentionally produced or feigned. Symptoms do not count toward a diagnosis of Somatization Disorder if they are intentionally produced or feigned.

Differential Diagnosis for Undifferentiated Somatoform Disorder

Undifferentiated Somatoform Disorder must be differentiated from . . .	In contrast to Undifferentiated Somatoform Disorder, the other condition . . .
Somatization Disorder	• Has a longer required duration (i.e., several years versus 6 months) and requires multiple and varied symptoms. Undifferentiated Somatoform Disorder is not diagnosed if the unexplained physical complaints are better accounted for by Somatization Disorder.
Factitious Disorder, Malingering	• Is characterized by symptoms that are intentionally produced or feigned. Undifferentiated Somatoform Disorder is not diagnosed if the unexplained physical complaints are intentionally produced or feigned.
Major Depressive Disorder, Anxiety Disorders, Adjustment Disorders, Sexual Dysfunctions, Sleep Disorders	• Includes physical complaints as associated features that need not be diagnosed separately. Undifferentiated Somatoform Disorder is not diagnosed if the unexplained physical complaints are better accounted for by another mental disorder.
Conversion Disorder, Pain Disorder, Sexual Dysfunction	• Is characterized by a specific physical complaint (e.g., pain, neurological deficit, sexual dysfunction). Undifferentiated Somatoform Disorder is not diagnosed if the criteria are met for one of these three disorders.

Differential Diagnosis for Conversion Disorder

Conversion Disorder must be differentiated from . . .	In contrast to Conversion Disorder, the other condition . . .
Occult neurological or other general medical conditions, Substance-Induced Disorders	• Fully accounts for the deficits involving voluntary motor or sensory functioning. Conversion Disorder can be diagnosed only if, after appropriate investigation, the symptom or deficit cannot be fully explained by a general medical condition or by the direct effects of a substance.
Pain Disorder, Sexual Dysfunction	• Is restricted to pain or sexual symptoms. Conversion Disorder is not diagnosed if the symptom is limited to pain or sexual dysfunction.
Somatization Disorder	• Includes in addition at least four pain symptoms, two gastrointestinal symptoms, and one sexual symptom. Conversion Disorder is not diagnosed if the symptom occurs exclusively during the course of Somatization Disorder.
Hypochondriasis	• Is characterized by a focus on the "serious disease" underlying the pseudoneurological symptoms.
Dissociative Disorders	• Involves neurological functions (e.g., memory, consciousness) other than voluntary motor or sensory functioning.
Factitious Disorder, Malingering	• Is characterized by symptoms that are intentionally produced or feigned. Conversion Disorder is not diagnosed if the symptoms are intentionally produced or feigned.

Differential Diagnosis for Pain Disorder

Pain Disorder must be differentiated from . . .	In contrast to Pain Disorder, the other condition . . .
Pain Disorder Associated With a General Medical Condition	• Is characterized by the absence of psychological factors that are judged to have a major role in the onset, exacerbation, or maintenance of the pain.
Somatization Disorder	• Requires multiple symptoms in addition to pain and a duration of at least several years. Pain Disorder Associated With Psychological Factors is not diagnosed if criteria are also met for Somatization Disorder.
Dyspareunia	• Is restricted to pain during sexual intercourse. Pain Disorder is not diagnosed if the pain meets the criteria for Dyspareunia.
Conversion Disorder	• Is characterized by deficits in voluntary motor or sensory functioning other than pain.
Other mental disorders (e.g., Anxiety Disorders, Psychotic Disorders)	• Includes pain as an associated feature that need not be diagnosed separately. Pain Disorder is not diagnosed if the pain is better accounted for by a Mood, Anxiety, or Psychotic Disorder.
Factitious Disorder, Malingering	• Is characterized by symptoms that are intentionally produced or feigned. Pain Disorder is not diagnosed if the pain is intentionally produced or feigned.

Differential Diagnosis for Hypochondriasis

Hypochondriasis must be differentiated from . . .	In contrast to Hypochondriasis, the other condition . . .
General medical condition	• Fully accounts for the physical symptoms.
Body Dysmorphic Disorder	• Is characterized by a focus on an imagined defect in physical appearance. Hypochondriasis is not diagnosed if the concern is restricted to appearance.
Somatization Disorder, Undifferentiated Somatoform Disorder, Conversion Disorder, Pain Disorder	• Is characterized by physical symptoms, but there is no preoccupation with the idea that one has a serious underlying disease.
Specific Phobia of contracting a disease	• Is characterized by a fear that one might contract a disease rather than a fear that one already has the disease.
Psychotic Disorders	• Is characterized by beliefs that are of delusional intensity. Hypochondriasis is not diagnosed if the belief is of delusional intensity.
Other mental disorders	• May include concerns about health as an associated feature that does not warrant a separate diagnosis. Hypochondriasis is not diagnosed if the preoccupation is better accounted for by Generalized Anxiety Disorder, Obsessive-Compulsive Disorder, Panic Disorder, a Major Depressive Episode, Separation Anxiety, or another Somatoform Disorder.
Expectable concerns about a general medical condition	• Includes worries that are realistic given the seriousness of the individual's medical status.

Differential Diagnosis for Body Dysmorphic Disorder

Body Dysmorphic Disorder must be differentiated from . . .	In contrast to Body Dysmorphic Disorder, the other condition . . .
Normal concerns about appearance	• Does not involve concerns that are excessively time consuming or that cause marked distress or impairment.
Eating Disorders	• Is characterized by concerns that are limited to body shape and weight. Body Dysmorphic Disorder is not diagnosed if the preoccupation is better accounted for by an Eating Disorder.
Gender Identity Disorder	• Includes concerns limited to primary or secondary sexual characteristics. Body Dysmorphic Disorder is not diagnosed if the preoccupation is better accounted for by Gender Identity Disorder.
Major Depressive Episode, Avoidant Personality Disorder, Social Phobia	• May include concerns about body appearance as an associated feature that does not warrant a separate diagnosis. Body Dysmorphic Disorder is not diagnosed if the preoccupation is better accounted for by another mental disorder.
Obsessive-Compulsive Disorder	• Includes intrusive thoughts and behaviors not limited to concerns about appearance.
Delusional Disorder, Somatic Type	• Is characterized by preoccupations that are held with delusional intensity. Body Dysmorphic Disorder may still be diagnosed even if the preoccupation is of delusional intensity.
Histrionic Personality Disorder, Narcissistic Personality Disorder	• Is characterized by a concern with appearance that does not involve specific defects.

Dissociative Disorders

Differential Diagnosis for Dissociative Amnesia

Dissociative Amnesia must be differentiated from . . .	In contrast to Dissociative Amnesia, the other condition . . .
Memory impairment in Delirium, Dementia, or Amnestic Disorder (either substance induced or due to a general medical condition); blackouts in Substance Intoxication	• Is characterized by gaps in memory that are not recoverable and is etiologically related to the direct physiological effect of a general medical condition or substance use.
Dissociative Fugue	• Requires unexpected travel and confusion about personal identity. Dissociative Amnesia is not diagnosed if the memory gaps occur exclusively during Dissociative Fugue states.
Dissociative Identity Disorder	• Includes the experience of alternate identities "taking control" of a person's behavior. Dissociative Amnesia is not diagnosed if the memory gaps occur exclusively during the course of Dissociative Identity Disorder.
Posttraumatic Stress Disorder or Acute Stress Disorder	• Requires the presence of an etiological extreme stressor and includes other characteristic symptoms (e.g., reexperiencing the trauma). Dissociative Amnesia is not diagnosed if the memory gaps occur exclusively during the course of Posttraumatic Stress Disorder or Acute Stress Disorder.

(continued)

Differential Diagnosis for
Dissociative Amnesia *(continued)*

Dissociative Amnesia must be differentiated from . . .	In contrast to Dissociative Amnesia, the other condition . . .
Somatization Disorder	• Includes multiple physical complaints. Dissociative Amnesia is not diagnosed if the memory gaps occur exclusively during the course of Somatization Disorder.
Malingering, Factitious Disorder	• Is characterized by amnesia that is feigned. Dissociative Amnesia is not diagnosed if the symptoms are feigned.
Age-Related Cognitive Decline	• Is related to normal aging.
Everyday memory loss, amnesia for dreams, amnesia for childhood experiences, posthypnotic amnesia	• Is not pathological.

Differential Diagnosis for
Dissociative Identity Disorder

Dissociative Identity Disorder must be differentiated from . . .	In contrast to Dissociative Identity Disorder, the other condition . . .
Mental Disorder Due to a General Medical Condition (e.g., complex partial seizures), Substance Intoxication or Withdrawal	• Is etiologically related to the direct physiological effect of a general medical condition or substance use.
Dissociative Amnesia, Dissociative Fugue, Depersonalization Disorder	• Is not characterized by the experience of having multiple distinct identities. Dissociative Amnesia and Dissociative Fugue are not diagnosed if symptoms occur exclusively during the course of Dissociative Identity Disorder.
Trance and possession states (Dissociative Disorder Not Otherwise Specified)	• Is characterized by the experience of external spirits "taking control."
Schizophrenia and other Psychotic Disorders	• Includes characteristic features (e.g., delusions, hallucinations, bizarre behavior, disorganized speech, negative symptoms).
Different mood states in Bipolar Disorder	• Includes Manic, Hypomanic, Mixed, or Major Depressive Episodes.
Borderline Personality Disorder	• Includes unstable identity but not the experience of having different personalities.
Malingering or Factitious Disorder	• Is characterized by symptoms that are feigned. Dissociative Identity Disorder is not diagnosed if the symptoms are feigned.

Sexual and Gender Identity Disorders

Differential Diagnosis for Primary Sexual Dysfunction

(Including Hypoactive Sexual Desire Disorder, Sexual Aversion Disorder, Female Sexual Arousal Disorder, Male Erectile Disorder, Orgasmic Disorder, Premature Ejaculation, Dyspareunia, and Vaginismus)

Primary Sexual Dysfunction must be differentiated from . . .	In contrast to Primary Sexual Dysfunction, the other condition . . .
Sexual Dysfunction Due to a General Medical Condition	• Requires the presence of an etiological general medical condition that completely accounts for the dysfunction. Primary Sexual Dysfunction is not diagnosed if the dysfunction is due exclusively to the direct physiological effects of a general medical condition. If psychological factors and a general medical condition are both contributory, the diagnosis is primary Sexual Dysfunction with the specifier Due to Combined Factors.
Substance-Induced Sexual Dysfunction	• Involves sexual dysfunction that is completely accounted for by medication side effects or a drug of abuse. Primary Sexual Dysfunction is not diagnosed if the dysfunction is due exclusively to the direct physiological effects of a substance.

(continued)

Differential Diagnosis for
Primary Sexual Dysfunction *(continued)*

Primary Sexual Dysfunction must be differentiated from . . .	In contrast to Primary Sexual Dysfunction, the other condition . . .
Sexual problems associated with another Axis I disorder (e.g., low sexual desire in the context of a Major Depressive Disorder)	• Involves sexual dysfunction occurring exclusively during the course of the Axis I condition that does not warrant independent clinical attention. Primary Sexual Dysfunction is not diagnosed if the dysfunction is better accounted for by another Axis I disorder.
Sexual problems associated with a relational problem	• Involves a Sexual Dysfunction that is often limited to a specific partner (situational) and is characterized by an exacerbation when the relational problem is worse. In some situations, both may be diagnosed together.

Differential Diagnosis for Paraphilias

(Including Exhibitionism, Fetishism, Frotteurism, Pedophilia, Sexual Masochism, Sexual Sadism, Transvestic Fetishism, and Voyeurism)

Paraphilias must be differentiated from . . .	In contrast to a Paraphilia, the other condition . . .
Nonpathological use of sexual fantasies, behaviors, or objects	• Does not cause clinically significant distress or impairment, is typically not obligatory for sexual functioning, and involves only consenting partners.
Sexual behavior resulting from a decrease in judgment, social skills, or impulse control related to another mental disorder (e.g., Manic Episode, Dementia, Schizophrenia)	• Is typically not an individual's preferred or obligatory pattern, occurs exclusively during the course of the mental disorder, often has a later age at onset, and is accompanied by the characteristic features of the mental disorder (e.g., cognitive impairment, delusions).

Differential Diagnosis for Gender Identity Disorder

Gender Identity Disorder must be differentiated from . . .	In contrast to Gender Identity Disorder, the other condition . . .
Nonconformity to stereotypic sex-role behavior	• Does not involve a profound disturbance in one's sense of maleness or femaleness and is not accompanied by significant distress or impairment.
Transvestic Fetishism	• Is characterized by cross-dressing for the purpose of sexual excitement and does not involve a profound disturbance in one's sense of maleness or femaleness.
Congenital intersex condition (e.g., androgen insensitivity syndrome, congenital adrenal hyperplasia)	• Is characterized by ambiguous genitalia (or other intersex manifestations). Gender Identity Disorder is not diagnosed concurrently with a physical intersex condition.

Eating Disorders

Differential Diagnosis for Anorexia Nervosa

Anorexia Nervosa must be differentiated from . . .	In contrast to Anorexia Nervosa, the other condition . . .
Weight loss in general medical conditions (e.g., neoplasms, infections, metabolic or endocrine conditions)	• Lacks requirement for distortion of body image and intense fear of getting fat; is often accompanied by loss of appetite; and includes signs, symptoms, or laboratory findings characteristic of the general medical condition.
Bulimia Nervosa	• Does not require low weight. Bulimia Nervosa can be diagnosed only at times when criteria are not met for Anorexia Nervosa. When criteria are met for both, Anorexia Nervosa, Binge-Eating/Purging Type is diagnosed.
Weight loss in Depressive Disorders	• Lacks requirement for intense fear of getting fat and includes the presence of characteristic features (e.g., depressed mood, loss of interest).
Unusual eating behavior in Schizophrenia	• Lacks requirement for intense fear of getting fat, is not characterized by low weight, and includes characteristic features (e.g., delusions, hallucinations, disorganized speech).
Food obsessions or compulsions in Obsessive-Compulsive Disorder	• Lacks requirement for intense fear of getting fat, is not characterized by low weight, and includes obsessions and compulsions that are not limited to thoughts or behaviors concerning weight, eating, or food.

(continued)

Differential Diagnosis for
Anorexia Nervosa *(continued)*

Anorexia Nervosa must be differentiated from . . .	In contrast to Anorexia Nervosa, the other condition . . .
Avoidance of eating in public in Social Phobia	• Lacks requirement for intense fear of getting fat and is not characterized by low weight.
Distortion of body image in Body Dysmorphic Disorder	• Lacks requirement for intense fear of getting fat and is not characterized by low weight.

Differential Diagnosis for Bulimia Nervosa

Bulimia Nervosa must be differentiated from . . .	In contrast to Bulimia Nervosa, the other condition . . .
Vomiting or diarrhea in general medical conditions or with excessive substance use	• Is due to the direct physiological effects of the general medical condition or substance use.
Binge eating in Anorexia Nervosa	• Requires weight below 85% of expected. Anorexia Nervosa, Binge-Eating/Purging Type, is diagnosed instead of Bulimia Nervosa if the binge eating occurs exclusively during the course of the Anorexia Nervosa.
Overeating in Depressive Disorders	• Does not require binges or inappropriate compensatory mechanisms and includes characteristic features (e.g., depressed mood, loss of interest).
Binge eating in Borderline Personality Disorder	• Does not require inappropriate compensatory mechanisms or overconcern with body shape and weight and includes characteristic features (e.g., self-mutilation, unstable relationships).
Eating Disorder Not Otherwise Specified (proposed category: binge-eating disorder)	• Is characterized by binge eating in the absence of the regular use of inappropriate compensatory mechanisms to counteract the effects of binge eating.

Sleep Disorders

Differential Diagnosis for Primary Insomnia

Primary Insomnia must be differentiated from . . .	In contrast to Primary Insomnia, the other condition . . .
Normal short sleepers	• Is not accompanied by difficulty falling asleep or fatigue, concentration problems, or irritability occurring during the day.
Daytime fatigue in Primary Hypersomnia	• Is not accompanied by difficulty falling asleep or maintaining sleep. Primary Hypersomnia is not diagnosed if the hypersomnia is better accounted for by insomnia.
Insomnia with Circadian Rhythm Sleep Disorder	• Is related to a "night-owl" or "starling" sleep pattern, jet lag, or shift work. Primary Insomnia is not diagnosed if the sleep disturbance occurs exclusively during Circadian Rhythm Sleep Disorder.
Sleep interruptions in Breathing-Related Sleep Disorder	• Is characterized by nighttime symptoms (e.g., loud snoring, breathing pauses) and physical examination and polysomnography findings. Primary Insomnia is not diagnosed if the sleep disturbance occurs exclusively during a Breathing-Related Sleep Disorder.
Sleep interruptions associated with Parasomnias	• Has a predominant complaint of nightmares, sleep terrors, or sleepwalking. Primary Insomnia is not diagnosed if the sleep disturbance occurs exclusively during a Parasomnia.

(continued)

Differential Diagnosis for Primary Insomnia (continued)

Primary Insomnia must be differentiated from . . .	In contrast to Primary Insomnia, the other condition . . .
Insomnia Related to Another Mental Disorder (e.g., Major Depressive Disorder, Schizophrenia)	• Occurs exclusively during the course of the other mental disorder. Insomnia Related to Another Mental Disorder is diagnosed instead of Primary Insomnia if the insomnia occurs exclusively during another mental disorder *and* is sufficiently severe to warrant independent clinical attention.
Insomnia that is an associated feature of another disorder and does not warrant a separate diagnosis	• Occurs exclusively during the course of the other mental disorder and does not warrant independent clinical attention.
Sleep Disorder Related to a General Medical Condition, Insomnia Type	• Requires the presence of an etiological general medical condition. Primary Insomnia is not diagnosed if the sleep disturbance is due to the direct physiological effects of a general medical condition.
Substance-Induced Sleep Disorder, Insomnia Type	• Is due to the direct physiological effects of a substance. Primary Insomnia is not diagnosed if the sleep disturbance is due to a substance.

Differential Diagnosis for Primary Hypersomnia

Primary Hypersomnia must be differentiated from . . .	In contrast to Primary Hypersomnia, the other condition . . .
Normal long sleepers	• Has no excessive daytime sleepiness or sleep drunkenness.
Inadequate amount of nocturnal sleep	• Results from inadequate sleep duration (e.g., fewer than 7 hours).
Daytime fatigue resulting from Primary Insomnia	• Is a consequence of difficulty maintaining or initiating sleep. Primary Insomnia takes precedence when symptoms of both insomnia and daytime fatigue are present.
Narcolepsy	• Is characterized by irresistible sleep attacks and specific polysomnography findings. Primary Hypersomnia is not diagnosed if the sleep disturbance occurs exclusively during the course of Narcolepsy.
Daytime sleepiness in Breathing-Related Sleep Disorder	• Is characterized by specific nighttime symptoms (e.g., loud snoring, breathing pauses) and physical examination and polysomnography findings. Primary Hypersomnia is not diagnosed if the sleep disturbance occurs exclusively during the course of Breathing-Related Sleep Disorder.
Daytime fatigue with Circadian Rhythm Sleep Disorder	• Is related to a "night-owl" or "starling" sleep pattern, jet lag, or shift work. Primary Hypersomnia is not diagnosed if the sleep disturbance occurs exclusively during the course of Circadian Rhythm Sleep Disorder.

(continued)

Differential Diagnosis for
Primary Hypersomnia *(continued)*

Primary Hypersomnia must be differentiated from . . .	In contrast to Primary Hypersomnia, the other condition . . .
Daytime fatigue associated with Parasomnias	• Has a predominant complaint of nightmares, sleep terrors, or sleep-walking. Primary Hypersomnia is not diagnosed if the sleep disturbance occurs exclusively during the course of a Parasomnia.
Hypersomnia Related to Another Mental Disorder (e.g., Major Depressive Disorder, Schizophrenia)	• Occurs exclusively during the course of the other mental disorder. Hypersomnia Related to Another Mental Disorder is diagnosed instead of Primary Hypersomnia if the hypersomnia occurs exclusively during another mental disorder and is sufficiently severe to warrant independent clinical attention.
Hypersomnia that is an associated feature of another disorder and does not warrant a separate diagnosis	• Occurs exclusively during the course of the other mental disorder and does not warrant independent clinical attention.
Sleep Disorder Related to a General Medical Condition, Hypersomnia Type	• Requires the presence of an etiological general medical condition. Primary Hypersomnia is not diagnosed if the sleep disturbance is due to the direct physiological effects of a general medical condition.
Substance-Induced Sleep Disorder, Hypersomnia Type	• Is due to the direct physiological effects of a substance. Primary Hypersomnia is not diagnosed if the sleep disturbance is due to a substance.

Impulse-Control Disorders

Differential Diagnosis for
Intermittent Explosive Disorder

Intermittent Explosive Disorder must be differentiated from aggressive behavior in . . .	In contrast to Intermittent Explosive Disorder, the other condition . . .
Substance Intoxication or Withdrawal	• Is due to the direct physiological effects of a substance. Intermittent Explosive Disorder is not diagnosed if aggressive behavior is due to a substance.
Delirium or Dementia (substance-induced or due to a general medical condition)	• Includes characteristic symptoms (e.g., memory impairment, impaired attention) and requires the presence of an etiological general medical condition or substance use. Intermittent Explosive Disorder is not diagnosed if aggressive behavior is part of Delirium or Dementia.
Personality Change Due to a General Medical Condition, Aggressive Type	• Requires presence of an etiological general medical condition. Intermittent Explosive Disorder is not diagnosed if aggressive behavior is better accounted for by a Personality Change Due to a General Medical Condition, Aggressive Type.
Conduct Disorder or Antisocial Personality Disorder	• Is characterized by a pattern of antisocial behavior. Intermittent Explosive Disorder is not diagnosed ifaggressive behavior is better accounted for by Conduct or Antisocial Personality Disorder.

(continued)

Differential Diagnosis for Intermittent Explosive Disorder (continued)

Intermittent Explosive Disorder must be differentiated from aggressive behavior in . . .	In contrast to Intermittent Explosive Disorder, the other condition . . .
Other mental disorders (e.g., Schizophrenia, Manic Episode, Oppositional Defiant Disorder, Borderline Personality Disorder)	• Includes other characteristic symptoms (e.g., delusions, elevated mood). Intermittent Explosive Disorder is not diagnosed if aggressive behavior is better accounted for by another mental disorder.
Aggressive behavior not attributable to a mental disorder	• Is motivated by political or religious belief, revenge, monetary gain, thrill seeking, or other reason not related to a mental disorder.

Differential Diagnosis for Kleptomania

Kleptomania must be differentiated from . . .	In contrast to Kleptomania, the other condition . . .
Ordinary acts of theft or shoplifting	• Is motivated by gain, peer approval, or rebellion, and there is a lack of tension/pleasure related to the theft.
Malingering	• Involves feigning to avoid prosecution.
Conduct Disorder or Antisocial Personality Disorder	• Is characterized by a more general pattern of antisocial behavior. Kleptomania is not diagnosed if stealing is better accounted for by Conduct Disorder or Antisocial Personality Disorder.
Episodes of stealing related to other mental disorders (e.g., Schizophrenia, Manic Episode, Dementia, Borderline Personality Disorder)	• Includes other characteristic symptoms (e.g., delusions, elevated mood). Kleptomania is not diagnosed if stealing is better accounted for by a Manic Episode.

Differential Diagnosis for Pyromania

Pyromania must be differentiated from . . .	In contrast to Pyromania, the other condition . . .
Other motives for fire setting (e.g., profit, revenge)	• Lacks tension/pleasure related to fire setting.
Developmental experimentation in childhood (e.g., playing with matches)	• Is restricted to childhood or adolescence and is not associated with a buildup and release of tension.
Conduct Disorder or Antisocial Personality Disorder	• Is characterized by a more general pattern of antisocial behavior. Pyromania is not diagnosed if fire setting is better accounted for by Conduct Disorder or Antisocial Personality Disorder.
Fire setting related to psychotic symptoms or impaired judgment in other mental disorders (e.g., Schizophrenia, Manic Episode, Dementia, Borderline Personality Disorder, Mental Retardation, Substance Intoxication)	• Includes other characteristic symptoms (e.g., delusions, elevated mood, cognitive impairment) of the other mental disorder. Pyromania is not diagnosed if fire setting is in response to a delusion or hallucination, is a result of impaired judgment (e.g., in Dementia, Mental Retardation, or Substance Intoxication), or is better accounted for by a Manic Episode.

Differential Diagnosis for Pathological Gambling

Pathological Gambling must be differentiated from . . .	In contrast to Pathological Gambling, the other condition . . .
Professional gambling	• Is characterized by discipline and limited risk taking and is intended to be a source of income.
Social gambling	• Usually occurs among friends and is characterized by limited time spent on gambling and limited risk taking.
Manic Episode	• Involves episodes of characteristic symptoms (e.g., flight of ideas) that persist at times when the individual is not gambling. Pathological Gambling is not diagnosed if the gambling behavior is better accounted for by a Manic Episode.

Differential Diagnosis for Trichotillomania

Trichotillomania must be differentiated from . . .	In contrast to Trichotillomania, the other condition . . .
General medical condition	• Fully accounts for the hair loss. Trichotillomania is not diagnosed if the hair pulling is due to a general medical condition.
Obsessive-Compulsive Disorder	• Is characterized by behavior that is performed in response to an obsession or according to rules that must be applied rigidly. Trichotillomania is not diagnosed if the hair pulling is better accounted for by Obsessive-Compulsive Disorder.
Schizophrenia or other Psychotic Disorders	• Is characterized by hair pulling in response to delusions or hallucinations. Trichotillomania is not diagnosed if the hair pulling is better accounted for by a Psychotic Disorder.
Stereotypic Movement Disorder	• Involves repetitive behaviors other than (or in addition to) hair pulling.
Factitious Disorder	• Is motivated by the desire to assume the sick role.

Adjustment Disorder

Differential Diagnosis for Adjustment Disorder

Adjustment Disorder must be differentiated from . . .	In contrast to Adjustment Disorder, the other condition . . .
All other specified mental disorders	• Is characterized by a specific symptom pattern and does not require that the symptoms occur in response to a stressor (except Posttraumatic Stress Disorder and Acute Stress Disorder). Adjustment Disorder is not diagnosed if the symptoms meet criteria for a specific Axis I disorder or if the symptoms are merely an exacerbation of an Axis II disorder.
Posttraumatic or Acute Stress Disorder	• Requires that the stressor be extreme and includes characteristic symptoms of intrusive thoughts, avoidance, dissociation, and physiological arousal.
Not Otherwise Specified categories (e.g., Depressive Disorder Not Otherwise Specified)	• Is diagnosed only when the criteria are not met for any specified DSM-IV disorder (including Adjustment Disorder).
Bereavement	• Is characterized by a reaction to the loss of a loved one that is in keeping with what would be expected. Adjustment Disorder can be diagnosed if the symptoms are in excess of what is expected.
Nonpathological reactions to stress	• Is characterized by symptoms that are within what would be expected given the nature of the stressor and that do not lead to clinically significant impairment.

Personality Disorders

Differential Diagnosis for Paranoid Personality Disorder

Paranoid Personality Disorder must be differentiated from . . .	In contrast to Paranoid Personality Disorder, the other condition . . .
Delusional Disorder, Persecutory Type; Schizophrenia, Paranoid Type; Mood Disorder With Psychotic Features	• Is characterized by a period of persistent psychotic symptoms. To give an additional diagnosis of Paranoid Personality Disorder, the Personality Disorder must have been present before the onset of psychotic symptoms and must persist when the psychotic symptoms are in remission.
Personality Change Due to a General Medical Condition, Paranoid Type	• Is characterized by a change in personality related to the direct effects of a general medical condition.
Social discomfort and paranoid ideation in Schizotypal Personality Disorder	• Also includes symptoms such as magical thinking, unusual perceptual disturbances, and odd speech or behavior.
Strange and aloof behavior in Schizoid Personality Disorder	• Is not characterized by paranoid ideation.
Reacting to minor stimuli in Borderline Personality Disorder or Histrionic Personality Disorder	• Is not necessarily associated with pervasive suspiciousness.
Reluctance to confide in others in Avoidant Personality Disorder	• Is due to a fear of being embarrassed or found inadequate.
Suspiciousness or alienation in Narcissistic Personality Disorder	• Is characterized by fears of having imperfections or flaws revealed.

Differential Diagnosis for
Schizoid Personality Disorder

Schizoid Personality Disorder must be differentiated from . . .	In contrast to Schizoid Personality Disorder, the other condition . . .
Delusional Disorder, Schizophrenia, Mood Disorder With Psychotic Features	• Is characterized by a period of persistent psychotic symptoms. To give an additional diagnosis of Schizoid Personality Disorder, the Personality Disorder must have been present before the onset of psychotic symptoms and must persist when the psychotic symptoms are in remission.
Autistic Disorder, Asperger's Disorder	• Is characterized by more severely impaired social interactions and stereotyped behaviors and interests.
Personality Change Due to a General Medical Condition, Apathetic Type	• Is characterized by a change in personality related to the direct effects of a general medical condition.
Schizotypal Personality Disorder	• Is characterized by cognitive and perceptual disturbances in addition to the social isolation.
Paranoid Personality Disorder	• Is characterized by suspiciousness and paranoid ideation.
Avoidant Personality Disorder	• Is characterized by an active desire for relationships that is constrained by a fear of embarrassment or rejection.
Obsessive-Compulsive Personality Disorder	• May be characterized by social detachment related to devotion to work and discomfort with emotions rather than lack of capacity to form intimate relationships.

Differential Diagnosis for
Schizotypal Personality Disorder

Schizotypal Personality Disorder must be differentiated from . . .	In contrast to Schizotypal Personality Disorder, the other condition . . .
Delusional Disorder, Schizophrenia, Mood Disorder With Psychotic Features	• Is characterized by a period of persistent psychotic symptoms. To give an additional diagnosis of Schizotypal Personality Disorder, the Personality Disorder must have been present before the onset of psychotic symptoms and must persist when the psychotic symptoms are in remission.
Autistic Disorder, Asperger's Disorder	• Is characterized by more severely impaired social interactions and stereotyped behaviors and interests.
Communication Disorders	• Is characterized by greater severity of disturbance in language accompanied by compensatory efforts to communicate by other means (e.g., gestures).
Personality Change Due to a General Medical Condition, Paranoid Type	• Is characterized by a change in personality related to the direct effects of a general medical condition.
Social detachment in Paranoid Personality Disorder and Schizoid Personality Disorder	• Is characterized by the lack of cognitive or perceptual distortions or marked eccentricity or oddness.
Avoidant Personality Disorder	• Is characterized by an active desire for relationships that is constrained by a fear of embarrassment or rejection.

(continued)

Differential Diagnosis for Schizotypal Personality Disorder *(continued)*

Schizotypal Personality Disorder must be differentiated from . . .	In contrast to Schizotypal Personality Disorder, the other condition . . .
Suspiciousness or social withdrawal in Narcissistic Personality Disorder	• Is related to fears of having imperfections revealed.
Borderline Personality Disorder	• Is characterized by impulsive and manipulative behavior.
Transient schizotypal traits in adolescents	• Reflects transient emotional turmoil rather than an enduring Personality Disorder.

Differential Diagnosis for Antisocial Personality Disorder

Antisocial Personality Disorder must be differentiated from . . .	In contrast to Antisocial Personality Disorder, the other condition . . .
Isolated antisocial behavior due to substance use	• Is exclusively related to drug taking and is not part of a pattern of antisocial behavior that began in childhood.
Antisocial behavior occurring in Schizophrenia or a Manic Episode	• Is associated with the characteristic symptoms of these disorders and is not associated with preexisting Conduct Disorder. Antisocial Personality Disorder should not be diagnosed if the antisocial behavior occurs exclusively during the course of Schizophrenia or a Manic Episode.
Glibness, exploitativeness, and lack of empathy in Narcissistic Personality Disorder	• Is not characterized by impulsivity, aggressiveness, and a previous pattern of Conduct Disorder.
Superficial emotionality in Histrionic Personality Disorder	• Is not characterized by impulsivity, aggressiveness, and a previous pattern of Conduct Disorder.
Manipulative behavior in Borderline Personality Disorder	• Is not characterized by impulsivity, aggressiveness, and a previous pattern of Conduct Disorder.
Antisocial behavior in Paranoid Personality Disorder	• Is motivated by revenge rather than desire for gain.
Adult antisocial behavior	• Is not characterized by a long-standing pattern of antisocial behavior with onset in childhood or adolescence and other personality features.

Differential Diagnosis for Borderline Personality Disorder

Borderline Personality Disorder must be differentiated from . . .	In contrast to Borderline Personality Disorder, the other condition . . .
Histrionic Personality Disorder	• Is not characterized by self-destructiveness, angry disruptions in close relationships, and chronic feelings of deep emptiness and loneliness.
Paranoid ideation or illusions in Schizotypal Personality Disorder	• Is characterized by paranoid ideation that is less interpersonally reactive and less amenable to the provision of external structure and support.
Paranoid ideation or angry reactions to minor stimuli in Paranoid Personality Disorder and Narcissistic Personality Disorder	• Is characterized by relative stability of self-image and relative lack of self-destructiveness, impulsivity, and abandonment concerns.
Manipulative behavior in Antisocial Personality Disorder	• Is characterized by manipulative behavior motivated by a desire for power, profit, or material gain rather than a desire for nurturance.
Abandonment concerns in Dependent Personality Disorder	• Is characterized by a reaction to the threat of abandonment with increasing appeasement and submission and attempts to seek a replacement relationship to provide caregiving and support.
Personality Change Due to a General Medical Condition, Labile Type	• Is characterized by a change in personality related to the direct effects of a general medical condition.
Identity problem	• Is characterized by identity concerns that are related to a developmental phase and that are less severe.

Differential Diagnosis for Histrionic Personality Disorder

Histrionic Personality Disorder must be differentiated from . . .	In contrast to Histrionic Personality Disorder, the other condition . . .
Borderline Personality Disorder	• Is characterized by self-destructiveness, angry disruptions in close relationships, and identity disturbance.
Manipulative behavior in Antisocial Personality Disorder	• Is characterized by manipulative behavior motivated by a desire for profit, power, or material gain rather than a desire for nurturance.
Attention seeking in Narcissistic Personality Disorder	• Is characterized by a need for praise for being superior.
Dependent Personality Disorder	• Is characterized by excessive dependence on others for praise and guidance without the flamboyant emotions characteristic of Histrionic Personality Disorder.
Personality Change Due to a General Medical Condition, Disinhibited Type	• Is characterized by a change in personality related to the direct effects of a general medical condition.

Differential Diagnosis for
Narcissistic Personality Disorder

Narcissistic Personality Disorder must be differentiated from . . .	In contrast to Narcissistic Personality Disorder, the other condition . . .
Need for attention in Histrionic Personality Disorder	• Is related to a need for approval as opposed to a need for admiration.
Lack of empathy in Antisocial Personality Disorder	• Is characterized by impulsivity, aggression, and deceit and is less characterized by a need for admiration by others.
Need for attention in Borderline Personality Disorder	• Is characterized by instability in self-image, self-destructiveness, impulsivity, and abandonment concerns.
Perfectionism in Obsessive-Compulsive Personality Disorder	• Is characterized by striving to attain perfection and a belief that others cannot do things as well, as opposed to a belief that perfection has already been achieved.
Suspiciousness and social withdrawal in Schizotypal Personality Disorder and Paranoid Personality Disorder	• Is related to paranoid ideation as opposed to fears of imperfections or flaws being revealed.
Grandiosity in Manic or Hypomanic Episodes	• Occurs only during episodes of elevated mood.
Personality Change Due to a General Medical Condition, Labile Type	• Is characterized by a change in personality related to the direct effects of a general medical condition.

Differential Diagnosis for Avoidant Personality Disorder

Avoidant Personality Disorder must be differentiated from . . .	In contrast to Avoidant Personality Disorder, the other condition . . .
Avoidance in Panic Disorder With Agoraphobia	• Typically starts after the onset of Panic Attacks and may vary based on their frequency and intensity.
Feelings of inadequacy, hypersensitivity to criticism, and need for reassurance in Dependent Personality Disorder	• Is characterized by concerns about being taken care of as opposed to avoidance of humiliation or rejection.
Social isolation in Schizoid Personality Disorder and Schizotypal Personality Disorder	• Is characterized by contentment with the social isolation or even a preference for social isolation.
Reluctance to confide in others in Paranoid Personality Disorder	• Is motivated by fears that personal information will be used with malicious intent as opposed to fears of being embarrassed.
Personality Change Due to a General Medical Condition	• Is characterized by a change in personality related to the direct effects of a general medical condition.

Differential Diagnosis for
Dependent Personality Disorder

Dependent Personality Disorder must be differentiated from . . .	In contrast to Dependent Personality Disorder, the other condition . . .
Dependency consequent to an Axis I disorder or a general medical condition	• Occurs exclusively during the Axis I disorder or general medical condition and varies according to its severity.
Fears of abandonment in Borderline Personality Disorder	• Is characterized by a reaction to anticipated abandonment with feelings of emotional emptiness, rage, and demands.
Need for reassurance and approval in Histrionic Personality Disorder	• Is characterized by gregarious flamboyance with active demands for attention.
Avoidant Personality Disorder	• Is characterized by such a strong fear of humiliation and rejection that there is social withdrawal until the person is certain of being accepted.
Personality Change Due to a General Medical Condition	• Is characterized by a change in personality related to the direct effects of a general medical condition.

Differential Diagnosis for Obsessive-Compulsive Personality Disorder

Obsessive-Compulsive Personality Disorder must be differentiated from . . .	In contrast to Obsessive-Compulsive Personality Disorder, the other condition . . .
Obsessive-Compulsive Disorder	• Is characterized by the presence of true obsessions and/or compulsions.
Perfectionism in Narcissistic Personality Disorder	• Is characterized by a belief that perfection has already been achieved.
Lack of generosity in Antisocial Personality Disorder	• Is characterized by an indulgence of self as opposed to a miserly spending style toward both self and others.
Social detachment in Schizoid Personality Disorder	• Occurs in the context of a lack of capacity for intimacy as opposed to discomfort with emotion and excessive devotion to work.
Personality Change Due to a General Medical Condition	• Is characterized by a change in personality related to the direct effects of a general medical condition.

4

DSM-IV-TR Symptom Index

The symptom index is a quick and convenient overview that can help form the basis for your differential diagnosis. It has a very different point of departure from the DSM-IV-TR Differential Diagnosis Tables. The tables are organized syndromally just as is DSM-IV-TR. Each disorder is defined by a cluster of symptoms that frequently co-occurs and that shares aspects of course, family history, and treatment response. As with the decision trees in Chapter 2, the symptom index helps you go in the reverse direction—from symptom to syndrome. Some of the symptoms covered in this chapter have also served as the starting point for decision trees presented in this book. However, many more symptoms are included here to provide a more fine-grained depiction of the system than was possible with the decision trees.

This index is divided into three parts. The first is a table of contents indicating where to find a symptom in the index. Next the symptom index is presented, with the symptoms listed in alphabetical order. For each symptom, there is a list of the DSM-IV-TR disorders that should come to mind when formulating the differential diagnosis for that symptom. It should be noted that, in some cases, the symptom list refers to syndromes (e.g., Panic Attack, Major Depressive Episode, Dementia). In such situations, one should also refer to the "Syndrome Index" in the third part of this index for an expanded list of disorders that are associated with that syndrome and in turn with a particular symptom.

Symptom Index of Psychiatric Symptoms

Symptom Index Table of Contents

Psychiatric Symptom Index

Substance Intoxication/
Withdrawal

Anhedonia

Acute Stress Disorder
Adjustment Disorder With
Depressed Mood
Bereavement
Dysthymic Disorder
Major Depressive Episode
(see entry, p. 229)
Mixed Episode (see entry, p. 229)
Posttraumatic Stress Disorder
Schizoaffective Disorder
Schizoid Personality Disorder
Schizophrenia
Schizophreniform Disorder
Schizotypal Personality Disorder
Substance Intoxication/
Withdrawal

Antisocial Behavior

Adjustment Disorder With
Disturbance of Conduct
Adjustment Disorder With Mixed
Disturbance of Emotions and
Conduct
Adult Antisocial Behavior
Antisocial Personality Disorder
Borderline Personality Disorder
Child or Adolescent Antisocial
Behavior
Conduct Disorder
Delusional Disorder
Hypomanic Episode (see entry,
p. 230)
Intermittent Explosive Disorder
Kleptomania
Manic Episode (see entry, p. 229)

Mixed Episode (see entry, p. 229)
Personality Change Due to a
General Medical Condition
Pyromania
Schizoaffective Disorder
Schizophrenia
Schizophreniform Disorder
Substance Dependence or Abuse
Substance Intoxication

Anxiety

Acute Stress Disorder
Agoraphobia Without History of
Panic Disorder
Anxiety Disorder Due to a
General Medical Condition
Avoidant Personality Disorder
Body Dysmorphic Disorder
Borderline Personality Disorder
Delirium
Delusional Disorder
Dependent Personality Disorder
Generalized Anxiety Disorder
Hypochondriasis
Major Depressive Episode
(see entry, p. 229)
Obsessive-Compulsive Disorder
Panic Attacks (see entry, p. 230)
Posttraumatic Stress Disorder
Schizophrenia
Schizophreniform Disorder
Schizotypal Personality Disorder
Separation Anxiety Disorder
Social Phobia
Somatization Disorder
Specific Phobia
Substance-Induced Anxiety
Disorder

Substance Intoxication/
  Withdrawal

Apathy

Acute Stress Disorder
Bereavement
Cyclothymic Disorder
Delirium (see entry, p. 229)
Dementia (see entry, p. 229)
Dysthymic Disorder
Major Depressive Episode
  (see entry, p. 229)
Personality Change Due to a
  General Medical Condition
Posttraumatic Stress Disorder
Schizophrenia
Substance Intoxication/
  Withdrawal

Appetite Disturbance

Adverse Effect of Medication Not
  Otherwise Specified
Anorexia Nervosa
Bulimia Nervosa
Major Depressive Episode
  (see entry, p. 229)
Substance Intoxication/
  Withdrawal

Avoidance Behavior

Acute Stress Disorder
Agoraphobia Without History of
  Panic Disorder
Avoidant Personality Disorder
Delusional Disorder
Dependent Personality Disorder
Dysthymic Disorder
Major Depressive Episode
  (see entry, p. 229)

Obsessive-Compulsive Disorder
Panic Disorder With Agoraphobia
Paranoid Personality Disorder
Pervasive Developmental Disorders
Posttraumatic Stress Disorder
Schizoaffective Disorder
Schizoid Personality Disorder
Schizophrenia
Schizophreniform Disorder
Schizotypal Personality Disorder
Separation Anxiety Disorder
Sexual Aversion Disorder
Social Phobia
Specific Phobia

Binge Eating

Anorexia Nervosa
Borderline Personality Disorder
Bulimia Nervosa

Blunted/Flat/Constricted Affect

Acute Stress Disorder
Dementia
Dysthymic Disorder
Major Depressive Episode
  (see entry, p. 229)
Obsessive-Compulsive Personality
  Disorder
Personality Change Due to a
  General Medical Condition
Posttraumatic Stress Disorder
Schizoid Personality Disorder
Schizophrenia
Schizotypal Personality Disorder
Substance Intoxication/
  Withdrawal

Catatonia

Brief Psychotic Disorder
Catatonic Disorder Due to a
General Medical Condition
Major Depressive Episode
(see entry, p. 229)
Manic Episode (see entry, p. 229)
Mixed Episode (see entry, p. 229)
Neuroleptic-Induced Acute
Dystonia
Neuroleptic-Induced Parkinsonism
Neuroleptic Malignant Syndrome
Schizoaffective Disorder
Schizophrenia
Schizophreniform Disorder

Cross-Dressing

Gender Identity Disorder
Transvestic Fetishism

Decrease in Energy or Fatigue

Breathing-Related Sleep Disorder
Dementia (see entry, p. 229)
Dysthymic Disorder
Generalized Anxiety Disorder
Major Depressive Episode
(see entry, p. 229)
Narcolepsy
Parasomnias
Personality Change Due to a
General Medical Condition
Primary Hypersomnia
Primary Insomnia
Schizoaffective Disorder
Schizophrenia
Schizophreniform Disorder

Substance Intoxication/
Withdrawal
Undifferentiated Somatoform
Disorder

Delusions

Brief Psychotic Disorder
Delirium (see entry, p. 229)
Delusional Disorder
Dementia (see entry, p. 229)
Major Depressive Episode
(see entry, p. 229)
Manic Episode (see entry, p. 229)
Mixed Episode (see entry, p. 229)
Psychotic Disorder Due to a
General Medical Condition
Schizoaffective Disorder
Schizophrenia
Schizophreniform Disorder
Shared Psychotic Disorder
Substance-Induced Psychotic
Disorder
Substance Intoxication/
Withdrawal

Depersonalization or Derealization

Agoraphobia Without History of
Panic Disorder
Borderline Personality Disorder
Depersonalization Disorder
Dissociative Identity Disorder
Hallucinogen Persisting Perception
Disorder
Panic Attacks (see entry, p. 230)
Schizoaffective Disorder
Schizophrenia
Schizophreniform Disorder
Substance Intoxication

Depressed Mood

Adjustment Disorder With
   Depressed Mood
Adjustment Disorder With Mixed
   Anxiety and Depressed Mood
Bereavement
Brief Psychotic Disorder
Cyclothymic Disorder
Delusional Disorder
Dementia (see entry, p. 229)
Dysthymic Disorder
Eating Disorders
Major Depressive Episode
   (see entry, p. 229)
Mixed Episode (see entry, p. 229)
Obsessive-Compulsive Disorder
Panic Disorder
Posttraumatic Stress Disorder
Schizoaffective disorder
Schizophrenia
Schizophreniform Disorder
Substance Intoxication/
   Withdrawal

Disorganized Speech/ Incoherence

Brief Psychotic Disorder
Delirium (see entry, p. 229)
Dementia (see entry, p. 229)
Expressive Language Disorder
Manic Episode (see entry, p. 229)
Mixed Episode (see entry, p. 229)
Mixed Receptive-Expressive
   Language Disorder
Schizoaffective Disorder
Schizophrenia
Schizophreniform Disorder
Substance Intoxication/
   Withdrawal

Distractibility

Attention-Deficit/Hyperactivity
   Disorder
Delirium (see entry, p. 229)
Hypomanic Episode (see entry,
   p. 230)
Manic Episode (see entry, p. 229)
Mixed Episode (see entry, p. 229)
Schizoaffective Disorder
Schizophrenia
Schizophreniform Disorder
Substance Intoxication/
   Withdrawal

Elevated Mood/Euphoria

Cyclothymic Disorder
Delirium (see entry, p. 229)
Hypomanic Episode (see entry,
   p. 230)
Manic Episode (see entry, p. 229)
Mixed Episode (see entry, p. 229)
Substance-Induced Mood Disorder
Substance Intoxication/
   Withdrawal

Feigning of Symptoms

Factitious Disorder
Malingering

Flight of Ideas

Cyclothymic Disorder
Hypomanic Episode (see entry,
   p. 230)
Manic Episode (see entry, p. 229)
Mixed Episode (see entry, p. 229)
Substance-Induced Mood Disorder
Substance Intoxication

Grandiosity

Brief Psychotic Disorder
Delirium (see entry, p. 229)
Delusional Disorder
Dementia (see entry, p. 229)
Hypomanic Episode (see entry,
   p. 230)
Manic Episode (see entry, p. 229)
Mixed Episode (see entry, p. 229)
Mood Disorder Due to a General
   Medical Condition
Narcissistic Personality Disorder
Psychotic Disorder Due to a
   General Medical Condition
Schizoaffective Disorder
Schizophrenia
Schizophreniform Disorder
Substance-Induced Mood Disorder
Substance Intoxication

Grossly Disorganized Behavior

Brief Psychotic Disorder
Delirium (see entry, p. 229)
Dementia (see entry, p. 229)
Personality Change Due to a
   General Medical Condition
Schizoaffective Disorder
Schizophrenia
Schizophreniform Disorder
Substance-Induced Psychotic
   Disorder
Substance Intoxication/ Withdrawal

Hallucinations

Brief Psychotic Disorder
Delirium (see entry, p. 229)
Dementia (see entry, p. 229)

Hallucinogen Persisting
   Perception Disorder
Major Depressive Episode
   (see entry, p. 229)
Manic Episode (see entry, p. 229)
Mixed Episode (see entry, p. 229)
Psychotic Disorder Due to a
   General Medical Condition
Schizoaffective Disorder
Schizophrenia
Schizophreniform Disorder
Substance-Induced Psychotic
   Disorder
Substance Intoxication/
   Withdrawal

Hypersomnia

Adverse Effects of Medication
   Not Otherwise Specified
Breathing-Related Sleep Disorder
Circadian Rhythm Sleep Disorder
Delirium (see entry, p. 229)
Dysthymic Disorder
Hypersomnia Related to Another
   Mental Disorder
Major Depressive Episode
   (see entry, p. 229)
Narcolepsy
Parasomnias
Primary Hypersomnia
Primary Insomnia
Schizoaffective Disorder
Schizophrenia
Schizophreniform Disorder
Sleep Disorder Due to a General
   Medical Condition
Substance-Induced Sleep Disorder
Substance Intoxication/Withdrawal

Impaired Abstract Thinking

Delirium (see entry, p. 229)
Dementia (see entry, p. 229)
Major Depressive Episode
   (see entry, p. 229)
Mental Retardation
Schizoaffective Disorder
Schizophrenia
Schizophreniform Disorder
Schizotypal Personality Disorder
Substance Intoxication/Withdrawal

Impaired Judgment

Antisocial Personality Disorder
Attention-Deficit/Hyperactivity
   Disorder
Borderline Personality Disorder
Brief Psychotic Disorder
Conduct Disorder
Delirium (see entry, p. 229)
Delusional Disorder
Dementia (see entry, p. 229)
Major Depressive Episode
   (see entry, p. 229)
Manic Episode (see entry, p. 229)
Mental Retardation
Mixed Episode (see entry, p. 229)
Paranoid Personality Disorder
Personality Change Due to a
   General Medical Condition
Substance Intoxication/Withdrawal

Inability to Maintain Attention/ Poor Concentration

Acute Stress Disorder
Attention-Deficit/Hyperactivity
   Disorder

Cyclothymic Disorder
Delirium (see entry, p. 229)
Dysthymic Disorder
Generalized Anxiety Disorder
Hypomanic Episode (see entry,
   p. 230)
Major Depressive Episode
   (see entry, p. 229)
Manic Episode (see entry, p. 229)
Mixed Episode (see entry, p. 229)
Posttraumatic Stress Disorder
Schizoaffective Disorder
Schizophrenia
Schizophreniform Disorder
Substance Intoxication/
   Withdrawal

Increase in Social, Occupational, or Sexual Activity

Cyclothymic Disorder
Hypomanic Episode (see entry,
   p. 230)
Manic Episode (see entry, p. 229)
Mixed Episode (see entry, p. 229)
Personality Change Due to a
   General Medical Condition
Substance-Induced Mood Disorder
Substance Intoxication

Indecisiveness

Dementia (see entry, p. 229)
Dependent Personality Disorder
Dysthymic Disorder
Major Depressive Episode
   (see entry, p. 229)
Obsessive-Compulsive
   Personality Disorder
Schizoaffective Disorder

Schizophrenia
Schizophreniform Disorder

Indifferent to Feelings of Others

Antisocial Personality Disorder
Asperger's Disorder
Autistic Disorder
Childhood Disintegrative Disorder
Conduct Disorder
Narcissistic Personality Disorder
Paraphilias
Pathological Gambling
Rett's Disorder
Schizoaffective Disorder
Schizophrenia
Schizophreniform Disorder
Schizoid Personality Disorder
Schizotypal Personality Disorder
Substance Dependence

Indiscriminate Socializing

Cyclothymic Disorder
Dementia (see entry, p. 229)
Histrionic Personality Disorder
Hypomanic Episode (see entry, p. 230)
Manic Episode (see entry, p. 229)
Mixed Episode (see entry, p. 229)
Personality Change Due to a General Medical Condition
Reactive Attachment Disorder of Infancy or Early Childhood
Substance Intoxication

Insomnia

Acute Stress Disorder
Breathing-Related Sleep Disorder

Circadian Rhythm Sleep Disorder
Cyclothymic Disorder
Delirium (see entry, p. 229)
Dysthymic Disorder
Generalized Anxiety Disorder
Hypomanic Episode (see entry, p. 230)
Insomnia Due to a General Medical Condition
Insomnia Related to Another Mental Disorder
Major Depressive Episode (see entry, p. 229)
Manic Episode (see entry, p. 229)
Mixed Episode (see entry, p. 229)
Nightmare Disorder
Posttraumatic Stress Disorder
Primary Insomnia
Schizoaffective Disorder
Schizophrenia
Schizophreniform Disorder
Sleep Terror Disorder
Sleepwalking Disorder
Substance-Induced Sleep Disorder
Substance Intoxication/ Withdrawal

Interpersonal Exploitativeness

Antisocial Personality Disorder
Borderline Personality Disorder
Conduct Disorder
Cyclothymic Disorder
Factitious Disorder
Hypomanic Episode (see entry, p. 230)
Malingering
Manic Episode (see entry, p. 229)

Mixed Episode (see entry, p. 229)
Narcissistic Personality Disorder
Pathological Gambling
Substance Dependence/Abuse
Substance Intoxication

Irritability

Acute Stress Disorder
Antisocial Personality Disorder
Attention-Deficit/Hyperactivity
   Disorder
Borderline Personality Disorder
Conduct Disorder
Cyclothymic Disorder
Delusional Disorder
Dysthymic Disorder
Generalized Anxiety Disorder
Hypomanic Episode (see entry,
   p. 230)
Major Depressive Episode
   (see entry, p. 229)
Manic Episode (see entry, p. 229)
Mixed Episode (see entry, p. 229)
Pathological Gambling
Posttraumatic Stress Disorder
Schizoaffective Disorder
Schizophrenia
Schizophreniform Disorder
Substance Intoxication/
   Withdrawal

Labile Affect

Borderline Personality Disorder
Cyclothymic Disorder
Delirium (see entry, p. 229)
Dementia (see entry, p. 229)
Hypomanic Episode (see entry,
   p. 230)

Major Depressive Episode
   (see entry, p. 229)
Manic Episode (see entry, p. 229)
Mixed Episode (see entry, p. 229)
Personality Change Due to a
   General Medical Condition
Schizoaffective Disorder
Schizophrenia
Schizophreniform Disorder
Substance Intoxication/
   Withdrawal

Memory Impairment

Acute Stress Disorder
Adverse Effect of Medication
   Not Otherwise Specified
Amnestic Disorder (see entry,
   p. 229)
Conversion Disorder
Delirium (see entry, p. 229)
Dementia (see entry, p. 229)
Dissociative Amnesia
Dissociative Fugue
Dissociative Identity Disorder
Major Depressive Episode
   (see entry, p. 229)
Posttraumatic Stress Disorder
Somatization Disorder
Substance Intoxication/
   Withdrawal

Paranoid Ideation

Amnestic Disorder
Delirium (see entry, p. 229)
Delusional Disorder
Dementia (see entry, p. 229)
Paranoid Personality Disorder
Personality Change Due to a
   General Medical Condition

Schizoaffective Disorder
Schizophrenia
Schizophreniform Disorder
Schizotypal Personality Disorder
Substance Intoxication/
  Withdrawal

Persistent Identity Disturbance

Borderline Personality Disorder
Dissociative Fugue
Dissociative Identity Disorder
Identity Problem
Schizoaffective Disorder
Schizophrenia
Schizophreniform Disorder

Physical Complaint Without General Medical Explanation

Body Dysmorphic Disorder
Conversion Disorder
Delusional Disorder
Generalized Anxiety Disorder
Hypochondriasis
Major Depressive Episode
  (see entry, p. 229)
Mixed Episode (see entry,
  p. 229)
Pain Disorder
Panic Attacks (see entry, p. 230)
Schizoaffective Disorder
Schizophrenia
Schizophreniform Disorder
Separation Anxiety Disorder
Somatization Disorder
Undifferentiated Somatoform
  Disorder

Pressured Speech

Cyclothymic Disorder
Hypomanic Episode (see entry,
  p. 230)
Manic Episode (see entry, p. 229)
Mixed Episode (see entry, p. 229)
Schizoaffective Disorder
Schizophrenia
Schizophreniform Disorder
Substance Intoxication

Psychomotor Agitation/ Restlessness

Adverse Effects of Medication
  Not Otherwise Specified
Cyclothymic Disorder
Delirium (see entry, p. 229)
Dementia (see entry, p. 229)
Hypomanic Episode (see entry,
  p. 230)
Major Depressive Episode (see
  entry, p. 229)
Manic Episode (see entry, p. 229)
Medication-Induced Akathisia
Mixed Episode (see entry, p. 229)
Schizoaffective Disorder
Schizophrenia
Schizophreniform Disorder
Substance Intoxication/Withdrawal

Psychomotor Retardation

Adverse Effects of Medication
  Not Otherwise Specified
Catatonic Disorder Due to a
  General Medical Condition
Delirium (see entry, p. 229)
Dementia (see entry, p. 229)

Major Depressive Episode
(see entry, p. 229)
Mixed Episode (see entry, p. 229)
Neuroleptic-Induced Parkinsonism
Schizoaffective Disorder
Schizophrenia
Schizophreniform Disorder
Substance Intoxication/Withdrawal

Repeated Lying

Antisocial Personality Disorder
Conduct Disorder
Factitious Disorder
Malingering
Pathological Gambling
Substance Dependence/Abuse

Restricted Travel Away From Home

Agoraphobia Without History of
Panic Disorder
Avoidant Personality Disorder
Delusional Disorder
Major Depressive Episode
(see entry, p. 229)
Panic Disorder With Agoraphobia
Separation Anxiety Disorder
Shared Psychotic Disorder
Social Phobia
Specific Phobia

Self-Induced Vomiting

Anorexia Nervosa
Bulimia Nervosa
Factitious Disorder
With Predominantly Physical
Signs and Symptoms
Malingering

Self-Mutilating Behavior

Borderline Personality Disorder
Dissociative Identity Disorder
Factitious Disorder With
Predominantly Physical Signs
and Symptoms
Malingering
Mental Retardation
Pervasive Developmental
Disorders
Sexual Masochism
Stereotypic Movement Disorder
Substance Intoxication/
Withdrawal
Trichotillomania

Sexual Dysfunction

Adjustment Disorder
Dyspareunia
Dysthymic Disorder
Female Arousal Disorder
Hypoactive Sexual Desire
Disorder
Major Depressive Episode
(see entry, p. 229)
Male Erectile Disorder
Male/Female Orgasmic Disorder
Mixed Episode (see entry, p. 229)
Paraphilias
Premature Ejaculation
Relational Problem
Sexual Abuse
Sexual Aversion Disorder
Sexual Dysfunction Due to a
General Medical Condition
Substance-Induced Sexual
Dysfunction
Substance Intoxication/
Withdrawal
Vaginismus

Social Isolation

Asperger's Disorder
Autistic Disorder
Avoidant Personality Disorder
Childhood Disintegrative Disorder
Rett's Disorder
Schizoaffective Disorder
Schizoid Personality Disorder
Schizophrenia
Schizophreniform Disorder
Schizotypal Personality Disorder

Speech Difficulties

Asperger's Disorder
Autistic Disorder
Childhood Disintegrative Disorder
Conversion Disorder
Delirium (see entry, p. 229)
Dementia (see entry, p. 229)
Expressive Language Disorder
Mixed Receptive-Expressive
    Language Disorder
Phonological Disorder
Rett's Disorder
Schizoaffective Disorder
Schizophrenia
Schizophreniform Disorder
Stuttering
Substance Intoxication/
    Withdrawal
Tic Disorder

Suicidal Ideation/ Suicide Attempt

Adjustment Disorder
Borderline Personality Disorder
Brief Psychotic Disorder

Conduct Disorder
Delusional Disorder
Major Depressive Episode
    (see entry, p. 229)
Manic Episode (see entry, p. 229)
Mixed Episode (see entry, p. 229)
Pain Disorder
Posttraumatic Stress Disorder
Schizoaffective Disorder
Schizophrenia
Schizophreniform Disorder
Substance Intoxication/
    Withdrawal

Weight Gain

Adverse Effects of Medication
    Not Otherwise Specified
Dysthymic Disorder
Major Depressive Episode
    (see entry, p. 229)
Mixed Episode (see entry, p. 229)
Schizoaffective Disorder
Schizophrenia
Schizophreniform Disorder
Substance Intoxication/
    Withdrawal

Weight Loss

Anorexia Nervosa
Dysthymic Disorder
Hypomanic Episode
    (see entry, p. 230)
Major Depressive Episode (see
    entry, p. 229)
Manic Episode (see entry, p. 229)
Mixed Episode (see entry, p. 229)
Substance Intoxication

Syndrome Index

DSM-IV-TR includes definitions of several syndromes that occur across a number of different disorders. The differential diagnosis depends on the accompanying symptoms, course, and specific etiological factors (e.g., substance use, general medical condition).

Delirium

Delirium Due to a General Medical
   Condition
Delirium Due to Multiple Etiologies
Substance Intoxication Delirium
Substance Withdrawal Delirium

Dementia

Dementia Due to Creutzfeldt-
   Jakob Disease
Dementia Due to Head Trauma
Dementia Due to HIV Disease
Dementia Due to Huntington's
   Disease
Dementia Due to Multiple
   Etiologies
Dementia Due to Other General
   Medical Condition
Dementia Due to Parkinson's
   Disease
Dementia Due to Pick's Disease
Dementia of the Alzheimer's Type
Substance-Induced Persisting
   Dementia
Vascular Dementia

Amnestic Disorder

Amnestic Disorder Due to a
   General Medical Condition
Substance-Induced Persisting
   Amnestic Disorder

Major Depressive Episode

Bipolar I Disorder
Bipolar II Disorder
Delusional Disorder
Dementia With Depressed Mood
Major Depressive Disorder
Mood Disorder Due to a General
   Medical Condition
Schizoaffective Disorder
Schizophrenia
Substance-Induced Mood
   Disorder

Manic Episode

Bipolar I Disorder
Mood Disorder Due to a General
   Medical Condition
Schizoaffective Disorder
Substance-Induced Mood
   Disorder

Mixed Episode

Bipolar I Disorder
Mood Disorder Due to a General
   Medical Condition
Schizoaffective Disorder
Substance-Induced Mood
   Disorder

Hypomanic Episode

Bipolar II Disorder
Cyclothymic Disorder
Mood Disorder Due to a General
    Medical Condition
Substance-Induced Mood Disorder

Panic Attacks

Adjustment Disorder With Anxiety
Anxiety Disorder Due to a General
    Medical Condition

Obsessive-Compulsive Disorder
Panic Disorder With/Without
    Agoraphobia
Posttraumatic Stress Disorder
Separation Anxiety Disorder
Social Phobia
Specific Phobia
Substance-Induced Anxiety
    Disorder

Appendix

DSM-IV-TR Classification

NOS = Not Otherwise Specified.

An *x* appearing in a diagnostic code indicates that a specific code number is required.

An ellipsis (. . .) is used in the names of certain disorders to indicate that the name of a specific mental disorder or general medical condition should be inserted when recording the name (e.g., 293.0 Delirium Due to Hypothyroidism).

If criteria are currently met, one of the following severity specifiers may be noted after the diagnosis:

Mild
Moderate
Severe

If criteria are no longer met, one of the following specifiers may be noted:

In Partial Remission
In Full Remission
Prior History

Disorders Usually First Diagnosed in Infancy, Childhood, or Adolescence

MENTAL RETARDATION

Note: *These are coded on Axis II.*
317   Mild Mental Retardation
318.0 Moderate Mental Retardation
318.1 Severe Mental Retardation
318.2 Profound Mental Retardation
319   Mental Retardation, Severity Unspecified

LEARNING DISORDERS

315.00 Reading Disorder
315.1   Mathematics Disorder
315.2   Disorder of Written Expression
315.9   Learning Disorder NOS

MOTOR SKILLS DISORDER

315.4   Developmental Coordination Disorder

COMMUNICATION DISORDERS

315.31 Expressive Language Disorder
315.32 Mixed Receptive-Expressive Language Disorder
315.39 Phonological Disorder
307.0   Stuttering
307.9   Communication Disorder NOS

PERVASIVE DEVELOPMENTAL DISORDERS

299.00 Autistic Disorder
299.80 Rett's Disorder
299.10 Childhood Disintegrative Disorder
299.80 Asperger's Disorder
299.80 Pervasive Developmental Disorder NOS

ATTENTION-DEFICIT AND DISRUPTIVE BEHAVIOR DISORDERS

314.xx Attention-Deficit/ Hyperactivity Disorder
  .01   Combined Type
  .00   Predominantly Inattentive Type
  .01   Predominantly Hyperactive-Impulsive Type
314.9   Attention-Deficit/Hyper- activity Disorder NOS
312.xx Conduct Disorder
  .81   Childhood-Onset Type
  .82   Adolescent-Onset Type
  .89   Unspecified Onset
313.81 Oppositional Defiant Disorder
312.9   Disruptive Behavior Disorder NOS

FEEDING AND EATING DISORDERS OF INFANCY OR EARLY CHILDHOOD

307.52 Pica
307.53 Rumination Disorder
307.59 Feeding Disorder of Infancy or Early Childhood

TIC DISORDERS

307.23 Tourette's Disorder
307.22 Chronic Motor or Vocal Tic Disorder
307.21 Transient Tic Disorder
        Specify if: Single Episode/ Recurrent
307.20 Tic Disorder NOS

ELIMINATION DISORDERS

——.–   Encopresis
787.6   With Constipation and Overflow Incontinence

307.7   Without Constipation and Overflow Incontinence

307.6   Enuresis (Not Due to a General Medical Condition)
Specify type: Nocturnal Only/ Diurnal Only/Nocturnal and Diurnal

OTHER DISORDERS OF INFANCY, CHILDHOOD, OR ADOLESCENCE

309.21   Separation Anxiety Disorder
Specify if: Early Onset

313.23   Selective Mutism

313.89   Reactive Attachment Disorder of Infancy or Early Childhood
Specify type: Inhibited Type/ Disinhibited Type

307.3   Stereotypic Movement Disorder
Specify if: With Self-Injurious Behavior

313.9   Disorder of Infancy, Childhood, or Adolescence NOS

Delirium, Dementia, and Amnestic and Other Cognitive Disorders

DELIRIUM

293.0   Delirium Due to . . . *[Indicate the General Medical Condition]*

——.—   Substance Intoxication Delirium *(refer to Substance-Related Disorders for substance-specific codes)*

——.—   Substance Withdrawal Delirium *(refer to Substance-Related Disorders for substance-specific codes)*

——.—   Delirium Due to Multiple Etiologies *(code each of the specific etiologies)*

780.09   Delirium NOS

DEMENTIA

294.xx   Dementia of the Alzheimer's Type, With Early Onset *(also code 331.0 Alzheimer's disease on Axis III)*

.10   Without Behavioral Disturbance

.11   With Behavioral Disturbance

294.xx   Dementia of the Alzheimer's Type, With Late Onset *(also code 331.0 Alzheimer's disease on Axis III)*

.10   Without Behavioral Disturbance

.11   With Behavioral Disturbance

290.xx   Vascular Dementia

.40   Uncomplicated

.41   With Delirium

.42   With Delusions

.43   With Depressed Mood
Specify if: With Behavioral Disturbance

Code presence or absence of a behavioral disturbance in the fifth digit for Dementia Due to a General Medical Condition

0 = Without Behavioral Disturbance
1 = With Behavioral Disturbance

294.1x   Dementia Due to HIV Disease *(also code 042 HIV on Axis III)*

294.1x   Dementia Due to Head Trauma *(also code 854.00 head injury on Axis III)*

294.1x   Dementia Due to Parkinson's Disease *(also code 332.0 Parkinson's disease on Axis III)*

294.1x   Dementia Due to Huntington's Disease *(also code*

333.4 *Huntington's disease on Axis III)*

294.1x Dementia Due to Pick's Disease *(also code 331.1 Pick's disease on Axis III)*

294.1x Dementia Due to Creutzfeldt-Jakob Disease *(also code 046.1 Creutzfeldt-Jakob disease on Axis III)*

294.1x Dementia Due to . . . *[Indicate the General Medical Condition not listed above] (also code the general medical condition on Axis III)*

——.– Substance-Induced Persisting Dementia *(refer to Substance-Related Disorders for substance-specific codes)*

——.– Dementia Due to Multiple Etiologies *(code each of the specific etiologies)*

294.8 Dementia NOS

AMNESTIC DISORDERS

294.0 Amnestic Disorder Due to . . . *[Indicate the General Medical Condition]*
Specify if: Transient/Chronic

——.– Substance-Induced Persisting Amnestic Disorder *(refer to Substance-Related Disorders for substance-specific codes)*

294.8 Amnestic Disorder NOS

OTHER COGNITIVE DISORDERS

294.9 Cognitive Disorder NOS

Mental Disorders Due to a General Medical Condition Not Elsewhere Classified

293.89 Catatonic Disorder Due to . . . *[Indicate the General Medical Condition]*

310.1 Personality Change Due to . . . *[Indicate the General Medical Condition]*
Specify type: Labile Type/ Disinhibited Type/Aggressive Type/Apathetic Type/Paranoid Type/Other Type/Combined Type/Unspecified Type

293.9 Mental Disorder NOS Due to . . . *[Indicate the General Medical Condition]*

Substance-Related Disorders

The following specifiers apply to Substance Dependence as noted:

[a]With Physiological Dependence/ Without Physiological Dependence
[b]Early Full Remission/Early Partial Remission/Sustained Full Remission/ Sustained Partial Remission
[c]In a Controlled Environment
[d]On Agonist Therapy

The following specifiers apply to Substance-Induced Disorders as noted:

[I]With Onset During Intoxication/
[W]With Onset During Withdrawal

ALCOHOL-RELATED DISORDERS

Alcohol Use Disorders

303.90 Alcohol Dependence[a,b,c]
305.00 Alcohol Abuse

Alcohol-Induced Disorders

303.00 Alcohol Intoxication
291.81 Alcohol Withdrawal
Specify if: With Perceptual Disturbances
291.0 Alcohol Intoxication Delirium
291.0 Alcohol Withdrawal Delirium
291.2 Alcohol-Induced Persisting Dementia

291.1 Alcohol-Induced Persisting Amnestic Disorder

291.x Alcohol-Induced Psychotic Disorder

.5 With Delusions[I,W]

.3 With Hallucinations[I,W]

291.89 Alcohol-Induced Mood Disorder[I,W]

291.89 Alcohol-Induced Anxiety Disorder[I,W]

291.89 Alcohol-Induced Sexual Dysfunction[I]

291.89 Alcohol-Induced Sleep Disorder[I,W]

291.9 Alcohol-Related Disorder NOS

AMPHETAMINE (OR AMPHETAMINE-LIKE)–RELATED DISORDERS

Amphetamine Use Disorders

304.40 Amphetamine Dependence[a,b,c]

305.70 Amphetamine Abuse

Amphetamine-Induced Disorders

292.89 Amphetamine Intoxication
Specify if: With Perceptual Disturbances

292.0 Amphetamine Withdrawal

292.81 Amphetamine Intoxication Delirium

292.xx Amphetamine-Induced Psychotic Disorder

.11 With Delusions[I]

.12 With Hallucinations[I]

292.84 Amphetamine-Induced Mood Disorder[I,W]

292.89 Amphetamine-Induced Anxiety Disorder[I]

292.89 Amphetamine-Induced Sexual Dysfunction[I]

292.89 Amphetamine-Induced Sleep Disorder[I,W]

292.9 Amphetamine-Related Disorder NOS

CAFFEINE-RELATED DISORDERS

Caffeine-Induced Disorders

305.90 Caffeine Intoxication

292.89 Caffeine-Induced Anxiety Disorder[I]

292.89 Caffeine-Induced Sleep Disorder[I]

292.9 Caffeine-Related Disorder NOS

CANNABIS-RELATED DISORDERS

Cannabis Use Disorders

304.30 Cannabis Dependence[a,b,c]

305.20 Cannabis Abuse

Cannabis-Induced Disorders

292.89 Cannabis Intoxication
Specify if: With Perceptual Disturbances

292.81 Cannabis Intoxication Delirium

292.xx Cannabis-Induced Psychotic Disorder

.11 With Delusions[I]

.12 With Hallucinations[I]

292.89 Cannabis-Induced Anxiety Disorder[I]

292.9 Cannabis-Related Disorder NOS

COCAINE-RELATED DISORDERS

Cocaine Use Disorders

304.20 Cocaine Dependence[a,b,c]

305.60 Cocaine Abuse

Cocaine-Induced Disorders

292.89 Cocaine Intoxication
Specify if: With Perceptual Disturbances

292.0 Cocaine Withdrawal

292.81 Cocaine Intoxication Delirium

292.xx   Cocaine-Induced Psychotic
         Disorder
   .11   With Delusions[I]
   .12   With Hallucinations[I]
292.84   Cocaine-Induced Mood
         Disorder[I,W]
292.89   Cocaine-Induced Anxiety
         Disorder[I,W]
292.89   Cocaine-Induced Sexual
         Dysfunction[I]
292.89   Cocaine-Induced Sleep
         Disorder[I,W]
292.9   Cocaine-Related Disorder
         NOS

HALLUCINOGEN-RELATED DISORDERS

Hallucinogen Use Disorders
304.50   Hallucinogen Dependence[b,c]
305.30   Hallucinogen Abuse

Hallucinogen-Induced Disorders
292.89   Hallucinogen Intoxication
292.89   Hallucinogen Persisting
         Perception Disorder
         (Flashbacks)
292.81   Hallucinogen Intoxication
         Delirium
292.xx   Hallucinogen-Induced
         Psychotic Disorder
   .11   With Delusions[I]
   .12   With Hallucinations[I]
292.84   Hallucinogen-Induced
         Mood Disorder[I]
292.89   Hallucinogen-Induced
         Anxiety Disorder[I]
292.9   Hallucinogen-Related
         Disorder NOS

INHALANT-RELATED DISORDERS

Inhalant Use Disorders
304.60   Inhalant Dependence[b,c]
305.90   Inhalant Abuse

Inhalant-Induced Disorders
292.89   Inhalant Intoxication
292.81   Inhalant Intoxication
         Delirium
292.82   Inhalant-Induced Persisting
         Dementia
292.xx   Inhalant-Induced Psychotic
         Disorder
   .11   With Delusions[I]
   .12   With Hallucinations[I]
292.84   Inhalant-Induced Mood
         Disorder[I]
292.89   Inhalant-Induced Anxiety
         Disorder[I]
292.9   Inhalant-Related Disorder
         NOS

NICOTINE-RELATED DISORDERS

Nicotine Use Disorder
305.1   Nicotine Dependence[a,b]

Nicotine-Induced Disorder
292.0   Nicotine Withdrawal
292.9   Nicotine-Related Disorder
         NOS

OPIOID-RELATED DISORDERS

Opioid Use Disorders
304.00   Opioid Dependence[a,b,c,d]
305.50   Opioid Abuse

Opioid-Induced Disorders
292.89   Opioid Intoxication
         Specify if: With Perceptual
         Disturbances
292.0   Opioid Withdrawal
292.81   Opioid Intoxication
         Delirium
292.xx   Opioid-Induced Psychotic
         Disorder
   .11   With Delusions[I]
   .12   With Hallucinations[I]
292.84   Opioid-Induced Mood
         Disorder[I]

292.89 Opioid-Induced Sexual Dysfunction[I]

292.89 Opioid-Induced Sleep Disorder[I,W]

292.9 Opioid-Related Disorder NOS

PHENCYCLIDINE (OR PHENCYCLIDINE-LIKE)–RELATED DISORDERS

Phencyclidine Use Disorders
304.60 Phencyclidine Dependence[b,c]
305.90 Phencyclidine Abuse

Phencyclidine-Induced Disorders
292.89 Phencyclidine Intoxication
        Specify if: With Perceptual Disturbances
292.81 Phencyclidine Intoxication Delirium
292.xx Phencyclidine-Induced Psychotic Disorder
  .11   With Delusions[I]
  .12   With Hallucinations[I]
292.84 Phencyclidine-Induced Mood Disorder[I]
292.89 Phencyclidine-Induced Anxiety Disorder[I]
292.9 Phencyclidine-Related Disorder NOS

SEDATIVE-, HYPNOTIC-, OR ANXIOLYTIC-RELATED DISORDERS

Sedative, Hypnotic, or Anxiolytic Use Disorders
304.10 Sedative, Hypnotic, or Anxiolytic Dependence[a,b,c]
305.40 Sedative, Hypnotic, or Anxiolytic Abuse

Sedative-, Hypnotic-, or Anxiolytic-Induced Disorders
292.89 Sedative, Hypnotic, or Anxiolytic Intoxication

292.0 Sedative, Hypnotic, or Anxiolytic Withdrawal
        Specify if: With Perceptual Disturbances
292.81 Sedative, Hypnotic, or Anxiolytic Intoxication Delirium
292.81 Sedative, Hypnotic, or Anxiolytic Withdrawal Delirium
292.82 Sedative-, Hypnotic-, or Anxiolytic-Induced Persisting Dementia
292.83 Sedative-, Hypnotic-, or Anxiolytic-Induced Persisting Amnestic Disorder
292.xx Sedative-, Hypnotic-, or Anxiolytic-Induced Psychotic Disorder
  .11   With Delusions[I,W]
  .12   With Hallucinations[I,W]
292.84 Sedative-, Hypnotic-, or Anxiolytic-Induced Mood Disorder[I,W]
292.89 Sedative-, Hypnotic-, or Anxiolytic-Induced Anxiety Disorder[W]
292.89 Sedative-, Hypnotic-, or Anxiolytic-Induced Sexual Dysfunction[I]
292.89 Sedative-, Hypnotic-, or Anxiolytic-Induced Sleep Disorder[I,W]
292.9 Sedative-, Hypnotic-, or Anxiolytic-Related Disorder NOS

POLYSUBSTANCE-RELATED DISORDER
304.80 Polysubstance Dependence[a,b,c,d]

OTHER (OR UNKNOWN) SUBSTANCE–RELATED DISORDERS

Other (or Unknown) Substance Use Disorders

304.90 Other (or Unknown) Substance Dependence[a,b,c,d]

305.90 Other (or Unknown) Substance Abuse

Other (or Unknown) Substance–Induced Disorders

292.89 Other (or Unknown) Substance Intoxication
Specify if: With Perceptual Disturbances

292.0   Other (or Unknown) Substance Withdrawal
Specify if: With Perceptual Disturbances

292.81 Other (or Unknown) Substance–Induced Delirium

292.82 Other (or Unknown) Substance–Induced Persisting Dementia

292.83 Other (or Unknown) Substance–Induced Persisting Amnestic Disorder

292.xx Other (or Unknown) Substance–Induced Psychotic Disorder
.11   With Delusions[I,W]
.12   With Hallucinations[I,W]

292.84 Other (or Unknown) Substance–Induced Mood Disorder[I,W]

292.89 Other (or Unknown) Substance–Induced Anxiety Disorder[I,W]

292.89 Other (or Unknown) Substance–Induced Sexual Dysfunction[I]

292.89 Other (or Unknown) Substance–Induced Sleep Disorder[I,W]

292.9   Other (or Unknown) Substance–Related Disorder NOS

Schizophrenia and Other Psychotic Disorders

295.xx Schizophrenia

The following Classification of Longitudinal Course applies to all subtypes of Schizophrenia:

Episodic With Interepisode Residual Symptoms (*specify if:* With Prominent Negative Symptoms)/ Episodic With No Interepisode Residual Symptoms

Continuous (*specify if:* With Prominent Negative Symptoms)

Single Episode In Partial Remission (*specify if:* With Prominent Negative Symptoms)/Single Episode In Full Remission

Other or Unspecified Pattern

.30   Paranoid Type
.10   Disorganized Type
.20   Catatonic Type
.90   Undifferentiated Type
.60   Residual Type

295.40 Schizophreniform Disorder
Specify if: Without Good Prognostic Features/With Good Prognostic Features

295.70 Schizoaffective Disorder
Specify type: Bipolar Type/ Depressive Type

297.1   Delusional Disorder
Specify type: Erotomanic Type/ Grandiose Type/Jealous Type/ Persecutory Type/Somatic Type/ Mixed Type/Unspecified Type

298.8 Brief Psychotic Disorder
Specify if: With Marked Stressor(s)/Without Marked Stressor(s)/With Postpartum Onset
297.3 Shared Psychotic Disorder
293.xx Psychotic Disorder Due to . . . *[Indicate the General Medical Condition]*
  .81 With Delusions
  .82 With Hallucinations
——.– Substance-Induced Psychotic Disorder *(refer to Substance-Related Disorders for substance-specific codes)*
Specify if: With Onset During Intoxication/With Onset During Withdrawal
298.9 Psychotic Disorder NOS

Mood Disorders

Code current state of Major Depressive Disorder or Bipolar I Disorder in fifth digit:

1 = Mild
2 = Moderate
3 = Severe Without Psychotic Features
4 = Severe With Psychotic Features
Specify: Mood-Congruent Psychotic Features/Mood-Incongruent Psychotic Features
5 = In Partial Remission
6 = In Full Remission
0 = Unspecified

The following specifiers apply (for current or most recent episode) to Mood Disorders as noted:

[a]Severity/Psychotic/Remission Specifiers/[b]Chronic/[c]With Catatonic Features/[d]With Melancholic Features/[e]With Atypical Features/[f]With Postpartum Onset

The following specifiers apply to Mood Disorders as noted:

[g]With or Without Full Interepisode Recovery/ [h]With Seasonal Pattern/[i]With Rapid Cycling

DEPRESSIVE DISORDERS

296.xx Major Depressive Disorder
  .2x Single Episode[a,b,c,d,e,f]
  .3x Recurrent[a,b,c,d,e,f,g,h]
300.4 Dysthymic Disorder
Specify if: Early Onset/Late Onset
Specify: With Atypical Features
311 Depressive Disorder NOS

BIPOLAR DISORDERS

296.xx Bipolar I Disorder
  .0x Single Manic Episode[a,c,f]
Specify if: Mixed
  .40 Most Recent Episode Hypomanic[g,h,i]
  .4x Most Recent Episode Manic[a,c,f,g,h,i]
  .6x Most Recent Episode Mixed[a,c,f,g,h,i]
  .5x Most Recent Episode Depressed[a,b,c,d,e,f,g,h,i]
  .7 Most Recent Episode Unspecified[g,h,i]
296.89 Bipolar II Disorder[a,b,c,d,e,f,g,h,i]
Specify (current or most recent episode): Hypomanic/Depressed
301.13 Cyclothymic Disorder
296.80 Bipolar Disorder NOS
293.83 Mood Disorder Due to . . . *[Indicate the General Medical Condition]*
Specify type: With Depressive Features/With Major Depressive–Like Episode/With Manic Features/With Mixed Features
——.– Substance-Induced Mood Disorder *(refer to Substance-Related Disorders*

for substance-specific codes)
Specify type: With Depressive
Features/With Manic Features/
With Mixed Features
Specify if: With Onset During
Intoxication/With Onset During
Withdrawal

296.90   Mood Disorder NOS

Anxiety Disorders

300.01   Panic Disorder Without
Agoraphobia
300.21   Panic Disorder With
Agoraphobia
300.22   Agoraphobia Without History
of Panic Disorder
300.29   Specific Phobia
Specify type: Animal Type/
Natural Environment Type/
Blood-Injection-Injury Type/
Situational Type/Other Type
300.23   Social Phobia
Specify if: Generalized
300.3   Obsessive-Compulsive
Disorder
Specify if: With Poor Insight
309.81   Posttraumatic Stress Disorder
Specify if: Acute/Chronic
Specify if: With Delayed Onset
308.3   Acute Stress Disorder
300.02   Generalized Anxiety
Disorder
293.84   Anxiety Disorder Due
to . . . *[Indicate the General
Medical Condition]*
Specify if: With Generalized
Anxiety/With Panic Attacks/
With Obsessive-Compulsive
Symptoms
—.–   Substance-Induced Anxiety
Disorder *(refer to Substance-
Related Disorders for
substance-specific codes)*
Specify if: With Generalized

Anxiety/With Panic Attacks/
With Obsessive-Compulsive
Symptoms/With Phobic Symptoms
Specify if: With Onset
During Intoxication/With
Onset During Withdrawal

300.00   Anxiety Disorder NOS

Somatoform Disorders

300.81   Somatization Disorder
300.82   Undifferentiated
Somatoform Disorder
300.11   Conversion Disorder
Specify type: With Motor
Symptom or Deficit/With
Sensory Symptom or Deficit/
With Seizures or Convulsions/
With Mixed Presentation
307.xx   Pain Disorder
.80   Associated With
Psychological Factors
.89   Associated With Both
Psychological Factors and
a General Medical
Condition
Specify if: Acute/Chronic
300.7   Hypochondriasis
Specify if: With Poor Insight
300.7   Body Dysmorphic Disorder
300.82   Somatoform Disorder NOS

Factitious Disorders

300.xx   Factitious Disorder
.16   With Predominantly
Psychological Signs and
Symptoms
.19   With Predominantly
Physical Signs and
Symptoms
.19   With Combined Psychological and Physical
Signs and Symptoms
300.19   Factitious Disorder NOS

Dissociative Disorders

300.12   Dissociative Amnesia
300.13   Dissociative Fugue
300.14   Dissociative Identity Disorder
300.6   Depersonalization Disorder
300.15   Dissociative Disorder NOS

Sexual and Gender Identity Disorders

SEXUAL DYSFUNCTIONS

The following specifiers apply to all primary Sexual Dysfunctions:

> Lifelong Type/Acquired Type
> Generalized Type/Situational Type
> Due to Psychological Factors/Due to Combined Factors

Sexual Desire Disorders

302.71   Hypoactive Sexual Desire Disorder
302.79   Sexual Aversion Disorder

Sexual Arousal Disorders

302.72   Female Sexual Arousal Disorder
302.72   Male Erectile Disorder

Orgasmic Disorders

302.73   Female Orgasmic Disorder
302.74   Male Orgasmic Disorder
302.75   Premature Ejaculation

Sexual Pain Disorders

302.76   Dyspareunia (Not Due to a General Medical Condition)
306.51   Vaginismus (Not Due to a General Medical Condition)

Sexual Dysfunction Due to a General Medical Condition

625.8   Female Hypoactive Sexual Desire Disorder Due to . . . *[Indicate the General Medical Condition]*

608.89   Male Hypoactive Sexual Desire Disorder Due to . . . *[Indicate the General Medical Condition]*
607.84   Male Erectile Disorder Due to . . . *[Indicate the General Medical Condition]*
625.0   Female Dyspareunia Due to . . . *[Indicate the General Medical Condition]*
608.89   Male Dyspareunia Due to . . . *[Indicate the General Medical Condition]*
625.8   Other Female Sexual Dysfunction Due to . . . *[Indicate the General Medical Condition]*
608.89   Other Male Sexual Dysfunction Due to . . . *[Indicate the General Medical Condition]*
——.—   Substance-Induced Sexual Dysfunction *(refer to Substance-Related Disorders for substance-specific codes)*
         Specify if: With Impaired Desire/With Impaired Arousal/With Impaired Orgasm/With Sexual Pain
         Specify if: With Onset During Intoxication
302.70   Sexual Dysfunction NOS

PARAPHILIAS

302.4   Exhibitionism
302.81   Fetishism
302.89   Frotteurism
302.2   Pedophilia
         Specify if: Sexually Attracted to Males/Sexually Attracted to Females/Sexually Attracted to Both
         Specify if: Limited to Incest
         Specify type: Exclusive Type/Nonexclusive Type
302.83   Sexual Masochism

302.84   Sexual Sadism
302.3   Transvestic Fetishism
         Specify if: With Gender Dysphoria
302.82   Voyeurism
302.9   Paraphilia NOS

GENDER IDENTITY DISORDERS

302.xx   Gender Identity Disorder
   .6   in Children
   .85   in Adolescents or Adults
             Specify if: Sexually Attracted
             to Males/Sexually Attracted to
             Females/Sexually Attracted to
             Both/Sexually Attracted to Neither
302.6   Gender Identity Disorder
         NOS
302.9   Sexual Disorder NOS

Eating Disorders

307.1   Anorexia Nervosa
         Specify type: Restricting Type;
         Binge-Eating/Purging Type
307.51   Bulimia Nervosa
         Specify type: Purging Type/
         Nonpurging Type
307.50   Eating Disorder NOS

Sleep Disorders

PRIMARY SLEEP DISORDERS

Dyssomnias

307.42   Primary Insomnia
307.44   Primary Hypersomnia
         Specify if: Recurrent
347   Narcolepsy
780.59   Breathing-Related Sleep
         Disorder
307.45   Circadian Rhythm Sleep
         Disorder
         Specify type: Delayed Sleep
         Phase Type/Jet Lag Type/Shift
         Work Type/Unspecified Type
307.47   Dyssomnia NOS

Parasomnias

307.47   Nightmare Disorder
307.46   Sleep Terror Disorder
307.46   Sleepwalking Disorder
307.47   Parasomnia NOS

**SLEEP DISORDERS RELATED TO
ANOTHER MENTAL DISORDER**

307.42   Insomnia Related to . . .
         *[Indicate the Axis I or
         Axis II Disorder]*
307.44   Hypersomnia Related to . . .
         *[Indicate the Axis I or
         Axis II Disorder]*

OTHER SLEEP DISORDERS

780.xx   Sleep Disorder Due to . . .
         *[Indicate the General
         Medical Condition]*
   .52   Insomnia Type
   .54   Hypersomnia Type
   .59   Parasomnia Type
   .59   Mixed Type
——.—   Substance-Induced Sleep
         Disorder *(refer to Substance-
         Related Disorders for
         substance-specific codes)*
         Specify type: Insomnia Type/
         Hypersomnia Type/Parasomnia
         Type/Mixed Type
         Specify if: With Onset During
         Intoxication/With Onset During
         Withdrawal

Impulse-Control Disorders Not Elsewhere Classified

312.34   Intermittent Explosive
         Disorder
312.32   Kleptomania
312.33   Pyromania
312.31   Pathological Gambling
312.39   Trichotillomania
312.30   Impulse-Control Disorder
         NOS

Adjustment Disorders

309.xx   Adjustment Disorder
.0   With Depressed Mood
.24   With Anxiety
.28   With Mixed Anxiety and
            Depressed Mood
.3   With Disturbance of
            Conduct
.4   With Mixed Disturbance
            of Emotions and Conduct
.9   Unspecified
            Specify if: Acute/Chronic

Personality Disorders

Note: *These are coded on Axis II.*
301.0   Paranoid Personality Disorder
301.20   Schizoid Personality Disorder
301.22   Schizotypal Personality
           Disorder
301.7   Antisocial Personality Disorder
301.83   Borderline Personality
           Disorder
301.50   Histrionic Personality Disorder
301.81   Narcissistic Personality
           Disorder
301.82   Avoidant Personality
           Disorder
301.6   Dependent Personality
           Disorder
301.4   Obsessive-Compulsive
           Personality Disorder
301.9   Personality Disorder NOS

Other Conditions That May Be a Focus of Clinical Attention

PSYCHOLOGICAL FACTORS AFFECTING MEDICAL CONDITION
316   . . . *[Specified Psychological
           Factor] Affecting . . . [Indi-
           cate the General Medical
           Condition]*
           *Choose name based on
           nature of factors:*
           Mental Disorder Affecting
              Medical Condition
           Psychological Symptoms
              Affecting Medical
              Condition
           Personality Traits or Coping
              Style Affecting Medical
              Condition
           Maladaptive Health
              Behaviors Affecting
              Medical Condition
           Stress-Related Physiological
              Response Affecting
              Medical Condition
           Other or Unspecified Psy-
              chological Factors Affect-
              ing Medical Condition

MEDICATION-INDUCED MOVEMENT DISORDERS
332.1   Neuroleptic-Induced
           Parkinsonism
333.92   Neuroleptic Malignant
           Syndrome
333.7   Neuroleptic-Induced Acute
           Dystonia
333.99   Neuroleptic-Induced Acute
           Akathisia
333.82   Neuroleptic-Induced
           Tardive Dyskinesia
333.1   Medication-Induced
           Postural Tremor
333.90   Medication-Induced
           Movement Disorder
           NOS

OTHER MEDICATION-INDUCED DISORDER
995.2   Adverse Effects of
           Medication NOS

RELATIONAL PROBLEMS

V61.9	Relational Problem Related to a Mental Disorder or General Medical Condition
V61.20	Parent-Child Relational Problem
V61.10	Partner Relational Problem
V61.8	Sibling Relational Problem
V62.81	Relational Problem NOS

PROBLEMS RELATED TO ABUSE OR NEGLECT

V61.21	Physical Abuse of Child *(code 995.54 if focus of attention is on victim)*
V61.21	Sexual Abuse of Child *(code 995.53 if focus of attention is on victim)*
V61.21	Neglect of Child *(code 995.52 if focus of attention is on victim)*
—.—	Physical Abuse of Adult
V61.12	(if by partner)
V62.83	(if by person other than partner) *(code 995.81 if focus of attention is on victim)*
—.—	Sexual Abuse of Adult
V61.12	(if by partner)
V62.83	(if by person other than partner) *(code 995.83 if focus of attention is on victim)*

ADDITIONAL CONDITIONS THAT MAY BE A FOCUS OF CLINICAL ATTENTION

V15.81	Noncompliance With Treatment
V65.2	Malingering
V71.01	Adult Antisocial Behavior
V71.02	Child or Adolescent Antisocial Behavior
V62.89	Borderline Intellectual Functioning *Note: This is coded on Axis II.*
780.9	Age-Related Cognitive Decline
V62.82	Bereavement
V62.3	Academic Problem
V62.2	Occupational Problem
313.82	Identity Problem
V62.89	Religious or Spiritual Problem
V62.4	Acculturation Problem
V62.89	Phase of Life Problem

Additional Codes

300.9	Unspecified Mental Disorder (nonpsychotic)
V71.09	No Diagnosis or Condition on Axis I
799.9	Diagnosis or Condition Deferred on Axis I
V71.09	No Diagnosis on Axis II
799.9	Diagnosis Deferred on Axis II

Multiaxial System

Axis I	Clinical Disorders Other Conditions That May Be a Focus of Clinical Attention
Axis II	Personality Disorders Mental Retardation
Axis III	General Medical Conditions
Axis IV	Psychosocial and Environmental Problems
Axis V	Global Assessment of Functioning

Index of Decision Trees and Differential Diagnosis Tables

Decision Trees

Differential Diagnosis Tables